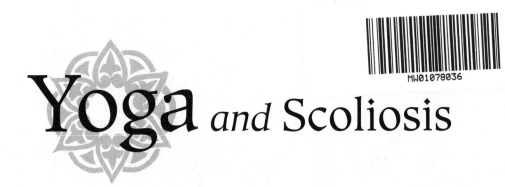

Yoga *and* Scoliosis

Yoga *and*

Scoliosis

A Journey to Health and Healing

MARCIA MONROE

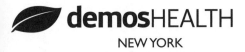

demosHEALTH

NEW YORK

Visit our Web site at www.demoshealth.com

ISBN: 978-1-9363-0302-1
E-book ISBN: 978-1-6170-5037-4

Acquisitions Editor: Noreen Henson
Compositor: Absolute Service, Inc.

Medical information provided by Demos Health, in the absence of a visit with a healthcare professional, must be considered as an educational service only. This book is not designed to replace a physician's independent judgment about the appropriateness or risks of a procedure or therapy for a given patient. Our purpose is to provide you with information that will help you make your own healthcare decisions.

The information and opinions provided here are believed to be accurate and sound, based on the best judgment available to the authors, editors, and publisher, but readers who fail to consult appropriate health authorities assume the risk of any injuries. The publisher is not responsible for errors or omissions. The editors and publisher welcome any reader to report to the publisher any discrepancies or inaccuracies noticed.

Library of Congress Cataloging-in-Publication Data

Monroe, Marcia.
  Yoga and scoliosis : a journey to health and healing / Marcia Monroe.
      p. ; cm.
  Includes bibliographical references and index.
  Summary: "Yoga and Scoliosis: A Journey to Health and Healing is intended to be a source of encouragement, knowledge, and healing for those who have scoliosis and need to treat it, but want to avoid braces and/or surgery. The book looks at scoliosis not as a pathological syndrome but as a spiritual, and metaphysical pattern that embraces the multiple dimensions of the spine (vertical, horizontal, and sagittal). It briefly covers the history and treatment modalities of scoliosis and discusses the development of the spine in the embryo. Yoga and Scoliosis also explores the complexities of the concept of alignment in the body, with the main part of the book showing how to address scoliosis with Iyengar yoga. Four chapters give instruction in yoga asanas for scoliosis, and another chapter discusses yoga practice in daily living. Finally there is an advanced yoga chapter that was developed by B. K. S. Inyengar"—Provided by publisher.
  ISBN 978-1-936303-02-1 (pbk.)
  I. Title.
  [DNLM: 1. Scoliosis—therapy. 2. Yoga. WE 735]
  LC classification not   assigned
  616.7'30642—dc23
                          2011030168

Printed in the United States of America by Bang Printing.
  14 15 / 5 4

*This book is dedicated to those seeking to understand
scoliosis through the depth of Yoga.
Yoga offers the possibility of finding answers
and sustaining hope for a better life inside of an
asymmetric body. It is possible.*

*My deepest dedication to my beloved teacher
BKS Iyengar, who gave me the gift to understand
the depth of embodiment and the wisdom of
acceptance through action.*

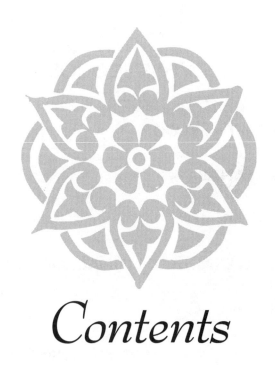

Contents

PART II

YOGA FOR SCOLIOSIS

PART III

ON DAILY LIFE

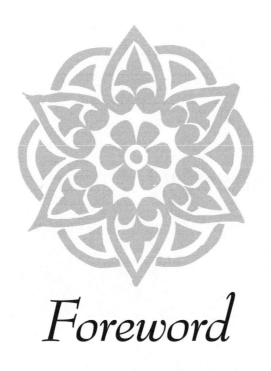

Foreword

I have read the synopsis of the book *Yoga and Scoliosis: A Journey to Health and Healing*. I have gone through the text along with the practical presentation and I feel that Marcia Monroe has done a good job. I am sure that her work will benefit many as they follow her presentation through her book for scoliosis, by correcting their defects with correct and proper alignment, and with the right method of support to get the maximum benefit with minimum effort.

Marcia Monroe first underwent correcting her own defects of the spine, and after experiencing the values of correct alignment, she undertook this work for fellow sufferers like her so that they might also benefit in minimizing or eradicating it totally.

I hope Marcia Monroe's work shall inspire those with scoliosis to make an attempt and live a lively life.

B.K.S. Iyengar

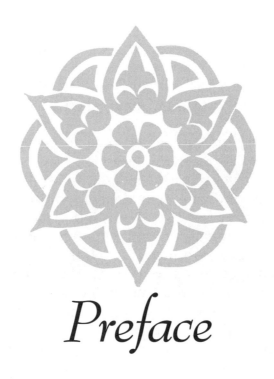

Preface

This book is called *Yoga and Scoliosis: A Journey to Health and Healing* because I have devoted my life's journey in searching for answers to the said condition. Being a survivor of idiopathic (meaning *of unknown cause*) scoliosis set me on the path of asking: What is this syndrome or pathology? Why and how does it manifest? What is its relationship to my expression, and how can it be improved?

My understanding of scoliosis has been highly influenced by the concept of motor developmental movement. I was introduced to the idea of ontogenesis—the development of an organism from embryo to adulthood—and to perceptual and motor developmental movement during my studies with Bonnie Bainbridge Cohen, the founder of the School for Body–Mind Centering. The theory is based on the principle that every cell has a memory and a developmental blueprint, and that it is possible to reteach the cells and, thus, learn new ways for the mind and body to work together.

My relationship with scoliosis began in my preadolescent years, from a very informal diagnosis by my aunt who noticed that my back was curved. She asked me to bend forward, as in the Adam's test used by physicians, and in doing so, she discovered one rib cage beginning to protrude. The next thing I knew, an orthopedic doctor's negative prognosis changed my life. He strongly recommended that I have my back straightened surgically.

However, I was a teenager and a dancer in my native country, Brazil, and I could not imagine having a metal rod in my back and undergoing the long process of uncertain recovery. I then made the choice not to undergo surgery, and after unsuccessful daily physical therapy and use of an orthopedic brace, I made the conscious choice to embark on my life's new mission: Embrace my scoliosis and explore it fully. Movement has always been my way of feeling my body, so I began by studying different forms of somatic movement therapies that related the body to the mind. Then I found yoga, and I have fully devoted myself to it since.

I was in New York City when I discovered yoga at Iyengar Institute, where I studied the Iyengar system with my first teacher, Mary Dunn, and eventually with Mr. Iyengar himself. As a system that involves physical, mental, and spiritual aspects, it fulfilled what I was searching for in terms of depth, embodiment, growth, constraint, restraint, being aware, and acting. From my very first class, I was introduced to concepts of stability and mobility, which are needed to connect with the asymmetric body and the internal body. I learned about the concept of constraints through the Yoga Sutras established by Shri Patanjali, the sage and grammarian of the late centuries BCE who codified yoga in aphorisms contained in four chapters. In the first chapter, called "Samadhi Pada," Patanjali defines yoga (yoga chitta vritti nirodha) as the restraint of one's fluctuations (thoughts); without restraint, there is no yoga. The Iyengar system of yoga is a practical tool for learning how to restrain and constrain the fluctuations from the body in order to unite it with the mind.

Yoga allows the brain to be reorganized in relation to the body through the practice of the asanas. One of my interests in scoliosis is how the nervous system learns and how it brings focus to each side of the body. In observing myself and others over the years, I have learned that in individuals with scoliosis, both of the sides learn differently. One side of the body learns and receives information, whereas the other is slower, and there tends to be greater sensitivity to the convex side. Through Iyengar yoga and specific asana sequences that emphasize symmetry and midline, I had glimpses of a centralized sensitivity, and began to focus on balancing and modifying both the concave and convex sides in my practice. Going from asymmetry to symmetry required tremendous practice, repetition, and willingness to learn, but I found that even when certain asanas were beyond my capability, the Iyengar system made it possible to work through challenging or painful movements through the innovative use of props and modified postures.

People often wonder whether yoga can improve scoliosis or decrease its curves. Younger students with scoliosis wonder whether they will one day have a straight spine. There is no single answer to this question because so many factors play into it. Physical makeup; genetics; personal history; lifestyle; the degree of the curve; and the student's willingness to learn, feel, participate, and improve all play into how successful the practice will be. In treating scoliosis, the spine must be considered from three dimensions: vertical, horizontal, and sagittal. Yoga provides students with a way of being sensitive to the asymmetries of the body and to deal with them intelligently. Each dimension is exercised—the vertical plane through lateral flexions that create side bends, the sagittal plane through flexion and extension patterns that create forward and backward motion, and the horizontal plane through rotations. Most importantly, however, treating scoliosis with yoga must be approached with commitment and discipline—and it can only be sustained if it is done with a sense of fun, curiosity, and enjoyment.

The information provided is this book is by no means intended to "cure" scoliosis or to perfectly explain the asanas and techniques. The information here is based on my lifelong studies and experience of how yoga has helped me, and I hope, in turn, will help you, too. However, this information is just a drop in the ocean; even the most experienced Yoga teachers seek to study and improve their practice every day.

Acknowledgments

Special thanks to my husband Arthur Monroe, for his solid and sustained support, love, and patience.

To B.K.S. Iyengar, the master of yoga, for his brilliant and profound method, and his son and daughter, Prashant Iyengar and Geeta Iyengar, for being the conduit of this precious and ancient legacy. I feel immense gratitude to the Iyengar family for helping me gain the objectivity to know the deep layers of myself through the science of yoga.

To Bonnie Bainbridge Cohen, for creating the method of Body-Mind Centering and for her pioneering and brilliant body of work in Embryology and psychosomatic awareness of body, mind, and soul.

To Moshe Feldenkrais, for his functional movement therapy method.

To all the students who have been my teachers.

To my yoga teachers and friends for their knowledge and help.

To my parents and family who have supported my search for knowledge of the spine up to this day.

My special thanks and gratitude to Noreen Henson for supporting the process of writing this book; without her this work would not have been possible.

ACKNOWLEDGMENTS

To Michael O'Connor for his work and help and to all of Demos Staff who have contributed to this project.

To my editors Robert Murray and Amanda Cushman for their immense support and help with the revisions.

To Cory Washburn for her marketing and her tremendous organizational skills and intelligence.

To our brilliant photographers, Virna Santolia and Luis Frota.

And finally, I would like to extend special gratitude to Doctor Loren Fishman for his participation in this book.

PART
I

INTRODUCTION

Introduction to Scoliosis

Dr. Loren Fishman, MD

Idiopathic scoliosis often begins in early puberty without specific cause, remains stable through most of life, and becomes painful in old age. Although it causes little disability up until this point, around the age of 60 or 70 years, the condition becomes increasingly severe and can restrict breathing. Often termed *degenerative scoliosis*, this condition can have grave medical consequences, especially if combined with other breathing and heart problems.

One simple fact of physics applies to scoliosis at any age: the greater the curve, the stronger the tendency for it to become more extreme. Therefore, treatment in the early stages is vital. However, to determine the best treatment for a condition, it is often useful to know the underlying cause.

NOTHING AS PRACTICAL AS A GOOD THEORY

The number of speculations about what causes scoliosis is inversely proportional to their certainty. Theories range from "handedness" to the location of the heart. The fact that nine-tenths of scoliosis cases occur in females lends credence to the genetic explanation. However, there is obviously something muscular about most cases of scoliosis; women have more delicate physiques that increase their susceptibility to muscular problems, and improving the spine's range of motion is known to deepen curves.

About 25 years ago, we were confronted with a frail, older woman with 113 degrees of an idiopathic, rotatory, thoracolumbar scoliosis: a tremendous C-curve. She also had asthma and mild cardiac abnormalities that, at once, made her ineligible for surgery and desperate for a cure. As luck would have it, she was a hospital administrator in a nearby state, and the facilities in her own institution had been tried and found wanting.

Sharing her desperation, and without a clue about the cause of her scoliosis, we reasoned, "Maybe we can't stop this process, but at least we can set up a contrary process that may be even stronger." We taught her static positions that we designed to strengthen the muscles on the bulging convex side.

Now, even though her spine was asymmetrical, there was a silver lining; her devoted daughter was a yoga teacher. Six months later, after predictably devout practice of the exercises we prescribed, we saw her again. All hands agreed; she was no worse. She had had so many x-rays in her life that we held off repeating them. She returned again after a little more than a year. This time, we looked at each other a little incredulously. She actually appeared to be straighter! After another 6 months, there was no question; her spine was coming back toward normal.

This time, none of us could resist checking things. We took an x-ray and were astounded by the results. The new scoliosis series showed a curve of 68 degrees! Spurred on by the good news, we kept on working. At different periods in her recovery, the postures we used changed.

Within the next 3 years, we essentially rectified this woman's posture and freed her breathing from the restrictive elements of her tilted and warped rib cage. When the progress we were making had slowed down nearly to a standstill, her curve was around 30 degrees. She retained this level of scoliosis for several years.

In the course of thinking about it, we developed our own theory of scoliosis: the human body, more so than other mammals, because of our upright posture, is a tensegrity structure—one that is held up by internal tension. Tensegrity is seen much in architecture, and is perhaps best exemplified by the Roman arches, in which weight from each side pillar presses against a trapezoidal keystone, holding it up.

The spine is a significantly more complex tensegrity structure than the Roman arch. Frei Otto, the prominent German architect, actually built a tower in the image of a stacked series of vertebrae. There are steel cables that run through them that are controlled by motors at the base. By differentially tightening and loosening them, the structure can be made to curve and twist in fairly authentic replication of human scoliosis.

Using the theory, we reasoned that the bulging side of a scoliosis curve, the convex side, might look larger and more developed because of the backward migrating ribs, but it was actually the weaker side. That side was being pulled harder than it was pulling, and stretched out of the position of normal, balanced support. Therefore, it was our job to devise, and the patient's job to undertake, asymmetrical positions that strengthened this seemingly overdeveloped side. In complex "S" curves, the task would be more challenging, requiring asymmetrical forces at different parts of the spine on opposite sides of the body. Fortunately, between side-support poses and twists, yoga offered many options. We will see this throughout the rest of the book.

Using this approach as a guideline, people actually started to reduce the curves as soon as 6 months after beginning the yoga exercises that follow. No one had reported such effects from exercise before. In fact, several studies had shown that exercise was useless, or worse. Previous efforts at conservative management had often concentrated on improving the spine's range of motion. Because gravity's force amplifies the muscular asymmetry already present in scoliosis, as the range of motion increases, gravity just takes up the slack and pulls the spine even further to the side and off of the midline. We explained our success by the fact that we strengthened the spine instead of increasing the range of motion. As muscular strength improved on the convex side, the muscles themselves increased the range of motion asymmetrically, permitting the spine to straighten while providing adequate support to keep it that way.

Over the years, we have had perhaps 75 or 100 patients with curves of various forms and complexity. We have always tried to adapt yoga or yoga-type poses to treat them, finding that yoga has distinct advantages over the other types of treatment that seemed reasonable.

Nothing we have said suggests that yoga is the only way to successfully treat scoliosis. How could anyone prove that? There are chiropractors, orthopedic surgeons, physical therapists, and other body workers that have had success. But what is it about yoga that renders it particularly suitable for ameliorating scoliosis?

Yoga May Strengthen the Muscles without Moving the Joints

Yoga postures make use of unusual positioning, in which your body's weight is supported by your arms, your hips, or the muscles of your torso. By pitting one muscle group against another, as in forward bends, each group—agonist and antagonist—is equally exerted and thereby strengthened.

Yoga Is Self-Administered

It can be done by oneself, every day, without elaborate equipment, even when traveling. A true alternative to an asymmetrical position can be reinforced on a consistent (and persistent) basis. Yoga's asanas have a definite aesthetic to them. Many yoga poses are like a catchy tune, and once done, are easily remembered.

Because Poses Are Held for Some Time, Yoga Works on the Tonic, Weight-Bearing Muscles Rather than the Quick-Acting Muscles that Are Chiefly Used for Manipulation

Whatever else yoga does, it retains the practitioner's position. These tonic, rather than clonic, activities of muscles are where the change to symmetry must take place. Yoga presents the kind of training that is needed to alter a life-long inclination toward scoliosis.

Yoga Is Essentially Free

After a short or spaced-out, intermittent period of learning, yoga is available to everyone.

Yoga Can Be Done until You Are Well over 100

Although prevention is preferable to cure, the older person with advancing scoliosis is in more and more immediate trouble than the youth. The ability to practice yoga very late in life allows it to be there when you need it.

Yoga Is Safe

Recent studies[1] find yoga injuries few and far between.

Yoga Is Versatile and Adaptable

People are smart. They adapt quite readily to exercises and find ways to do them while altering their usual posture and stance as little as possible. There are numerous occasions on which patients have returned after 2 weeks and showed us how they perform an exercise designed to ward off increasing lordosis, in a manner that increases lordosis. One must observe and update the asana when dealing with a wily species such as ourselves.

There is one other matter that we should consider. Because scoliosis is a medical condition, it should be monitored by a physician. This is helpful for judging what other conditions might be limiting the patient's ability to recover symmetry, such as radiculopathy (pinched nerve roots), hip or sacroiliac joint abnormalities, or neuromuscular or cerebrovascular conditions. Even anemia can limit a patient's ability to put a full effort into the asanas that are wisely prescribed.

In addition, the physician may help monitor the patients' progress, which inspires both the patient and the yoga therapist, helps the latter determine which poses are the most beneficial (or, let's face it, harmful), and may aid in directing more patients toward a yoga-based therapy that is beneficial, inexpensive, and has few unwanted and many desirable side effects.

One prime example of an asana that has proven helpful in treating scoliosis is vasisthasana. There are various versions from lying sideways (convex curve down) against a wall with forearm and hips on the floor and raising only the midsection and ribs of the concave side, to the classic pose itself.

But this is just to whet your appetite. Now, the time for sitting and reading may be past. Come on. There are curves just waiting to unwind.

[1.] L. M. Fishman, E. Saltonstall, and S. Genis, "Understanding and Preventing Yoga Injuries," *International Journal of Yoga Therapy* 19, no.1 (2009): 1–8.

2

Yoga

The translation in English for the Sanskrit word *yoga* is "to join, to unite." Yoga is a science that teaches the means of joining the body, the mind, and the human soul with the underlying creative force of the universe. Yoga literature speaks to the concept of awareness, as related to one's life force or energy, and is meant to derive from—and be present in—every cell of the body. In yoga practice, this means developing a keen awareness of your own body, to the point of *learning* both sides of the body in relation to themselves and your surroundings. By embracing this idea of self-discovery, you will gain knowledge and become deeply aware of the structure of your own body. This is the first step toward not only enhanced physical harmony, but also a strengthened connection of body, mind, and spirit.

In *Yoga Sutras of Patanjali*, which is thought to date to the fifth century BCE, the sage Patanjali codifies Yoga in four chapters or padas. In the second chapter, Patanjali lays out the practical steps, or eight "limbs" (Ashtanga Yoga), for the student of Yoga to attain freedom. They are classified as yamas (universal ethics), nyamas (personal ethics and observances), asanas (postures), pranayama (breath control), pratyahara (turning the senses inward), dharana (fixing the attention), and samadhi (communion).

This book focuses on asanas that are particularly useful for scoliosis, and touches briefly on the first steps of pranayama as it relates to the yoga postures (asanas). It follows the Iyengar tradition, because his methods provide ways for those with scoliosis to experience postures that might otherwise be impossible.

7

HOW TO USE THIS BOOK

Yoga and Scoliosis has been written to share the benefits of yoga as a science that provides physical, mental, and spiritual transformation and ways to decrease suffering. The sequences given in this book, unlike mechanical exercises or therapies that focus on the cause of the scoliosis only, view the entire person, and they are modifiable for each individual's condition. The underlying goal of this book is to emphasize the importance of learning about yourself, to understand the structure of your body, and to learn basic principles to work with scoliosis.

The modified yoga sequences suggested here will allow you to improve self-organization, to correct your posture, and to alleviate pain, stress, and fatigue. They are to be used as a resource to increase stability, proper alignment, energy, independence, and self-awareness. These sequences should be conducted under the guidance of a senior teacher, and with medical supervision.

The main intention of this book is to provide a way to find healing and freedom through embracing the scoliotic condition. Your willingness to learn and improve will open the door to hope. With this book, you will discover how to better live with scoliosis, and live a highly functional and experientially rich life.

GUIDELINES FOR PERSONAL AND GROUP PRACTICE

Personal practice is the most important time to learn, feel, and connect with yourself. Like a building, every asana has a foundation, the ground from which the rest of the body coordinates and lifts. The embodiment process—the full connection of mind and body—begins in understanding your curves along both sides. The understanding of how your body influences your mind and vice versa will allow you to gain intelligence and self-confidence, and take control of your practice.

If you are a beginner, you should work with a teacher before attempting the asanas on your own. A teacher, especially a senior teacher who has trained in the Iyengar tradition, can help you achieve the ideal alignment, as well as show you how to use props to create support. Once you have mastered the basics, you may consider practicing on your own.

SUGGESTIONS FOR PERSONAL AND GROUP PRACTICE

1. Establish a space for practice or teaching that supports the inner engagement of the mind. Ideally, it should be clean, quiet, and without distractions. Organize all the props in a suitable place, and when you finish the practice, put the props back so you can start fresh the next time. For scoliosis, it is imperative to have external organization, and that begins with the environment.
2. In a group class, let the teacher know if you are in pain, or if there is any other health condition. If you have a Harrington rod, it is important to tell the teacher where the fusion is, and to be extra conservative in the practice. Use enough props to avoid putting strain and pressure on the metal. The order of exercises will be tailored to your individual needs. As a suggestion, practice the standing postures with enough height

to elongate the torso without straining the spine. The supported forward extensions and hip flexions are to be performed in the concave phase only. Twists should be mild and done in a chair or well supported by blankets. The rope wall practice used in the Iyengar system can be very helpful to elongate the spine without strain. An example of rope wall use is supported rope adho mukha svanasana (dog pose with the wall rope on the upper thigh) followed by mild back extension and legs flat against the wall. Finish your practice with restorative asanas and mild inversions followed by savasana (the resting posture). Use imagery to create sensitivity within the unmovable areas. Have a physician approve your practice because many postures might be contraindicated. Work with a teacher who understands spinal fusions. Explore the standing postures with support, the hip flexions and supported forward extensions.

3. A restorative sequence starts on the floor with supported supine and prone postures and ends on the floor. By starting out on the floor, you will release extra tension, relieve fatigue, and gain more information about your body's asymmetries and the breath that will be useful as you sit and then stand. The floor, like a mirror, will act as a guide to self-learning and the proper correction.

4. Because scoliosis must be viewed three-dimensionally, each side must be modified according to your condition to end up in a symmetrical position.

5. Touch is a powerful learning tool for scoliosis. Use the information you gain through touch about the contour of the bones to determine what needs to lift, what is displaced, and what needs to move inward. In all the positions, distribute the body weight evenly between the right and left sides.

6. Work with the principle of traction—the mechanical stretching of the spine to straighten it—but know that even in stretched positions, the tendency is for the scoliosis to take over. The traction will offer space for self-correction. Props will also offer external traction, because when one area of the body is fixed, the opposite area lengthens.

7. Create length by using opposing actions.

8. Learn how to use the props as support for stabilization, elongation, and alignment. There are infinite ways to work with props, so be creative and remain stable. Learn how to feel the spine so as not to compress it. The proper height of the props will help to achieve the best position.

9. Work with the breath to expand and fill the side that is short and retracted, and to deflate or compact the side that feels expanded. Trade roles between sides.

10. Use props to support your body's asymmetry in any lying, sitting, or standing position. Both sides need support so that the chest can spread horizontally as well as vertically. As you grow to understand your body and yoga, decrease the height of the support. Finally, use the knowledge you gained from your studies to design your own forms of support.

11. Whenever modifying an asana from symmetry to asymmetry in order to work with both sides, always return to the symmetrical position at the finish.

12. Do not skip *savasana*. Support both sides of the spine in savasana so the chest can open and the breath can flow. Savasana, or the deep rest, is the time to integrate and assimilate and to quiet the nervous system from its constant tracking.

FINDING THE RIGHT PROPS FOR YOU

One of the many gifts that Mr. Iyengar has given to the West is the use of props as tools for better alignment. The props modify the asanas according to your needs, and give a person with scoliosis a sense of where they are in space. In addition, with the support of props, the organ system, instead of being obscure, becomes something you are conscious of.

B. K. S. Iyengar has created special ways to use straps and belts for various conditions. In the case of scoliosis, they support the shoulder blades, ribs, and pelvis and direct the movement of the skin counter to the scoliosis. These straps and belts act like a spinal brace that wraps the body without making it rigid, thereby providing a sense of containment that is needed in scoliosis.

Having scoliosis alters one's perception of positions in space, and the props offer external markers of organization. For this reason, it is important to arrange them symmetrically on your mat. The precision of their placement will allow you to remain oriented to where you are on the mat. Use external references, such as the edges of your mat and the lines on the floor, to help you arrange the props appropriately.

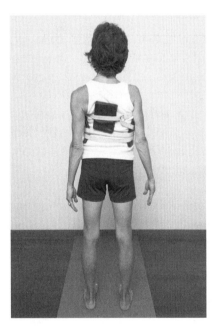 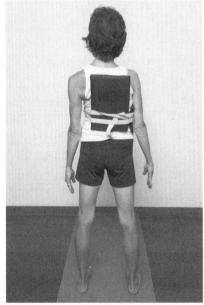 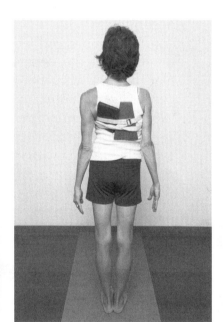

SUGGESTIONS FOR PROPS

- Mat with geometric lines to help midline and spatial orientation
- Several yoga blankets and cloths for feedback from both sides
- Blocks and pads, both thin and thick
- Belts of different shapes and sizes for traction and stabilization
- Wall ropes and single ropes for traction
- Wall, column, door, kitchen counter, yoga trestler (horse) for various standing and other postures
- Head wrap or bag to relax the eyes and nervous system
- Chairs, tables, benches, stools
- Tall stool for forward and backward extensions, twists, and support for the limbs
- Light plate weights or sandbags for skeletal proprioception to enhance normal levels of muscular tension and relax the nerves
- Mirror as a reference to improve alignment
- Physioball, 30–45 inches, for various asanas

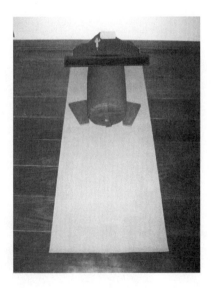
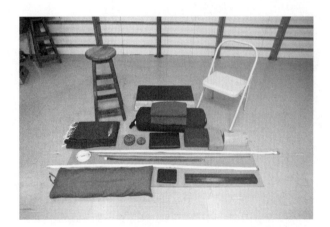

3

Concepts of Sequencing

A ny sequencing is to be supervised under the guidance of a teacher, tailored according to the individual's level, and, most importantly, her condition.

SEQUENCING A PRACTICE FOR SCOLIOSIS

What I suggest in the next chapters are modified asanas, based on my own experience and that of my students. The postures will be effective whether your scoliosis is idiopathic or non-idiopathic. Other scoliosis conditions can be treated with the understanding that the asanas work with each of the three-dimensional spine's planes (vertical, horizontal, and sagittal), and so all deformities are taken into account as a result. The key is that the sequence in which you perform yoga postures should be created for you individually, taking into account your history, etiology of the scoliosis, diagnosis, age, and familiarity with yoga. The sequence should include the various families of asanas and should take into account all three dimensions, with the aim of increasing length; improving proprioception and balance; stabilizing and strengthening the body; and most of all, arresting further progression of the scoliosis.

Sequencing from Ground to Standing

There are many ways to sequence a practice, depending on the student's experience, medical history, and age. As a rule, any sequence should not introduce harm, fatigue, or progression of the curves and should finish with the cooling restorative asanas followed by savasana. The resting time is very important for allowing the body to integrate the newly learned motions and recuperate from the effort.

The asanas mentioned in the subsequent text follow the natural human developmental pattern of lying down to standing. This does not mean that a sequence should always start on the floor, but rather that the ground offers the body the opportunity to learn: to retrace patterns and establish new ways to organize. The vast repertoire of yoga postures teaches the body how to differentiate and to integrate its concave and convex sides. Through practice you gain stability and mobility from the relationship of gravity to the body's resistance to gravity (antigravity).

The supine (on your back), prone (on your stomach), and side-lying postures provide proprioception (awareness of the position of your body in relation to its various parts, gravity, and space). The floor provides feedback on how the body lies and interacts, or not, with gravity. Even the simple act of lying down on the floor with the legs and arms extended, hands facing up, will inform you of your habitual posture. In standing, the wall can, like the floor, increase the proprioception of the back and body parts.

Learning where your asymmetries are from the supine and prone postures will guide you toward the ways in which you can best support your body. The lying positions release contracted areas and lower the high tension of the muscles that keep you upright. This makes lying down postures an excellent place for beginning students to develop awareness, and the place we will begin. After studying these positions, you can introduce props to align your body and begin to create balance between the two sides.

PART II

YOGA FOR SCOLIOSIS

Postures on the Floor

SUPINE POSTURES

Lying on the back

Evaluating your posture on the floor

Props

Yoga mat, wall.

Benefits

Lying flat on the floor engages the mind with the body, so it can discern the asymmetries and lower the tension of contracted muscles. Once you have discovered where these are, the next step is to find the proper support for the best alignment for the reclining postures.

Placement

Simply lie down and observe your contact with the floor.

What to Observe

- Extension of the legs: Which leg extends faster? Which seems to be longer? How do the backs of the legs touch the floor?
- Position of the feet: Do they tend to supinate (roll out) or pronate (roll in)?
- The space behind the knees: Does one knee tend to bend (flex) more than the other?
- Position of the thighs: Which thigh touches the floor and which comes away? Which one rolls to the side?
- Pelvis: Does one side of the hip bone (ilium) lift away from the floor and rotate toward the front of the body? Or does one side elevate toward the ribs? Is the pubic bone centered in relation to the navel, sternum, and nose?
  The pubic bone will reflect the asymmetry of the pelvis (lumbar curve).
- Back ribs: Which side collapses back and feels heavier? Which side lifts away from the floor and feels lighter?
- Front ribs: Which side of the upper thoracic ribs caves in and closes the chest? Which side of the chest puffs up? Which side of the lower ventral ribs protudes out and rotates and which side pulls down?
- Chest: Which side of the chest feels open or closed? Note the position of the chest bone in relation to the navel and nose. How does each shoulder blade touch the floor?
- Shoulders: On which side does the scapula (shoulder bone) move in and the back of the upper arm touch the floor (also called retraction)? On which side does the scapula move out and the back upper arm lift away (protraction)? Which shoulder moves toward the ear, and which one moves away from the ear?
- Arms: Which arm is closer to the body? Which arm is farther?

- Position of the hands: How do both hands establish contact with the floor?
- Neck: How much space is there between the back of the neck and the floor? Are both sides of the neck even? Which side feels longer?
- Head: How does the back of the head touch the floor? Does it tend to roll toward one side?
- Spine: How does the spine touch the floor? How do you feel your backbone? Which areas are heavy and which feel suspended and light? What is the length of the spine? How much space is there between the tailbone and the head? How much weight does each side of the body bear on the floor? Notice the spaces between the body and the floor. Which side feels longer? Which side feels compressed?
- Breath: How does the breath move through both sides?
- Notice the gaze. Are the eyes looking at the ceiling? Is one eye more active than the other?

In the beginning, it is particularly important to have a teacher evaluate you in this position. Teachers need to observe all the things mentioned previously and notice how the student lies in relation to the mat, the position of the limbs, head, neck, chest, and where the rolling is, the tilting, or the lack or abundance of space.

After observing the asymmetries, the next step is to figure out how to support the areas that feel suspended from the floor (concavities), how to lift the areas that are heavy on the floor, and to feel the relationship of the limbs and the center. There are infinite ways and strategies for using the props. The principle of the props is to lift the areas that sink, to create a relationship with the areas that feel suspended and retracted, to support both sides, and to create comfort.

Pay attention to your eyes. They will show you what is going on in the brain and in the nervous system, and this will be reflected in the temples, throat, neck, shoulders, skin, and breath.

The following are a few variations. As a general rule, the legs act on the lumbar spine and the arms on the upper thoracic and cervical spine. Therefore, adjustment to the individual scoliosis must be done accordingly to create the proper traction, elongation, and counter-rotation.

Please note that the following instructions are merely modifications of the full postures. For the complete instructions on performing the classic asanas in this book, please consult *Light on Yoga* by B. K. S. Iyengar.

SUPTA TADASANA: MOUNTAIN POSTURE ON THE FLOOR

Props

Mat, wall, blankets, small wooden wedges, pads to even the asymmetry of the shoulders, ribs, and pelvis. Blankets are used lengthwise and are folded to support both sides of the spine. An extra blanket can be placed horizontally to open and lift the chest.

Benefits

Supta tadasana, being a symmetric posture, helps in stabilizing the core as it brings midline (central) organization from the extension of the limbs. It offers stability within the asymmetric body. The front of the body (flexors) moves toward the back (extensors), and the spine stabilizes.

Placement

Place the mat with one end by the wall. Fold a blanket in a vertical shape that will support both ends of the spine (the tailbone and the back of the head). Sit in the center of it in dandasana (legs together and stretched out in front of you), with the feet together touching the wall. Bend both legs (moving forward to keep your feet on the wall), place the forearms on the floor, look up at the ceiling, and lie back. Press the feet on the wall as you slowly extend both legs; see whether one foot has less pressure or is losing contact with the wall, and whether one side tends to extend faster. If it does, inhibit the action by bending the legs again, moving closer to the wall, and restarting. Continue to press the feet on the wall and extend both legs. Lie with the arms alongside of the torso, palms facing each other.

Note

In cases of severe scoliosis and pain, spread the legs to the outer edge of the mat. This decentralized position will help the back to spread to the sides and will distribute the weight evenly throughout the body. Additional props such as blankets are used according to your curve and to support the back of the head. The main goal of the support is to lift the areas that collapse toward the floor and to support the areas that lift away from the floor. To avoid rotation on the hips and shoulders, small towels or pads can be placed on the outer edges of the area that rolls toward the floor.

In all the supine variations, if the lumbar spine lifts away from the floor, spread an extra blanket folded in half horizontally under the pelvis. In the case of a lumbar curve scoliosis, use pads to even the hip rotation (on the outer edge of the hip that collapses) and under the segment where the spinal curve is (convex side) to avoid further collapses.

You'll see me wearing belts and pads in the following pictures. The addition of belts and pads can be useful to stabilize the trunk and offer a counter-rotational force; however, their use must be taught and overseen by a senior teacher on an individual basis.

Not everyone needs extra props. Sometimes, lying without props is a great way to activate the muscles and coordinate them.

What to Do

Bring both legs together, and press your feet against the wall. Extend the legs and press the thighs toward the floor. Compact the outer hips (i.e., draw them together), lengthen the tailbone, and lift the pubic bone up. Rotate the upper arms as the hand supinates (palm facing up); press the back of the hands onto the floor, extend the fingers, and move the outer edge of the shoulder blades in. Move the shoulders away from the ears and spread the collarbones. Press the foot on your concave (short) side firmly against the wall to lengthen it, moving the hip away from the rib cage. Spread the ribs. Finally, press both feet evenly, and extend the legs and the sides of the body.

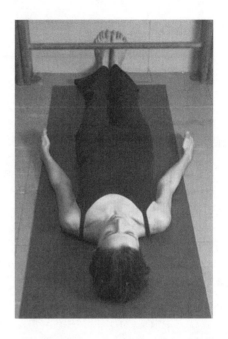

The position of the eyes and gaze will affect the position of the head and neck. Gaze at the ceiling with receptive eyes. Use the proper support for the head (up to two blankets).

If the setup is not appropriate, come up and reorganize the props. You might need extra blankets and pads. Both convex and concave sides should be supported.

Variation 1: With Blocks

Props

Mat, wall, blankets, three blocks, three belts for the legs, pads, and wooden wedges.

Benefits

The addition of the block helps to coordinate the limbs, induce internal rotation toward the midline, and provide stability and a sense of evenness.

What To Do

As your palms turn up, extend your arms, and roll your shoulders back and away from the ears with the outer portion of the shoulder blades moving in toward the spine (mainly on the convex side). As you press your feet, extend your legs and lengthen both sides of the trunk, maintaining the waist toward the floor.

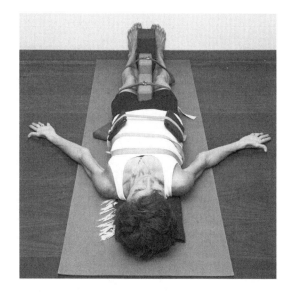

Fold a blanket length-wise to support both sides of the spine, and use pads to support the outer hips in order to prevent them from rolling. Finally, place wedges under the convex posterior ribs to lift the chest. Repeat the exercise as mentioned previously, but take one block and place it between your feet, place another block between the lower legs (shins), and a third block, the same size as the second, between the upper inner thighs. The inside of the legs will be in firm contact with the blocks.

If the blocks are not giving the sense of centeredness and stability, take three belts and loop each one around each block and the body part (feet, lower leg, and thighs). Alternate the directions of the belt loops. If the knees are moving inward (knock knees), place a small pad in between them. Ideally, a teacher will place the blocks and the belts. Extend the legs in this compacted position. The arms extend to the sides with the hands facing up.

Variation 2: Lifting the Arms

Props

Mat, wall, blanket, three blocks, two belts for legs.

Benefits

The action of lifting the arms over the head is a trajectory that will reveal the misalignments of the shoulders and how to correct them.

Placement

From supta tadasana, lift both arms up with the palm of the hands facing each other. Bring both arms up in line with the shoulders and perpendicular to the floor. Note whether the back of the arms and shoulders are touching the floor in this position. Now decentralize your arms and observe if this action has helped to create more width and broadening of the chest. Continue the motion of the arms over the head.

Note

Although the ideal alignment is to have the arms in a perpendicular line to the floor and over the shoulders for thoracic curves, this might be challenging for you. By moving the arms slightly out to the sides, you create space and experience the desired movement toward evenness.

What to do

Extend the legs and press the feet on the wall. As you lift both arms up toward the ceiling, bring both shoulders down toward the floor. Move the shoulder blades in toward the ribs (mainly on the convex side) and move the upper arm down to the floor. As you continue to move the arms over the head, press the feet against the wall, extend the legs, and bring both sides of the waist down toward the floor. Bring your arms in line with both shoulders.

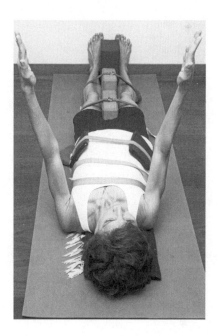

Continue the movement and extend both arms over the head. Synchronize both sides. The main point is to stabilize the arm in the socket, and to bring the shoulder blades in, the shoulders away from the ears, and the back of the arms down. Feel or look to see whether one arm is closer to the trunk and adjust accordingly. Pause in places of difficulty or if the shoulders lift away from the floor. It is important to lift both arms up symmetrically over the head, to extend the fingers and both elbows so they face each other, and to do the movement very slowly.

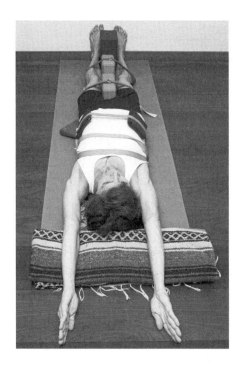

Variation 3: Holding a Block

Props

Mat, wall, three blocks, two blankets, three belts.

Benefits

The block will add resistance for the arms to elongate and firm the shoulder blades. The principle is to bring alignment to both sides, to lift the areas that collapse toward the floor, and to open the chest. From these observations, use the appropriate props to lift the drops and to lift the chest, as well as to reduce the concavities and rotations. If the chest is sagging, mainly because of the weight of the convex side, fold a blanket horizontally under the thoracic spine or place a wooden plank under the chest. Because of the over-developed convex rib cage, the shoulder blades lose their stability and feel disconnected from the spine, and the chest closes.

Placement

Repeat the actions of the previous posture, now holding a block between the hands. There will likely be a tendency for one side to move faster going up and down and for one shoulder to lift up faster. During these moments, go slower and reestablish the position of both shoulders. Control the movement by stabilizing the upper arm toward the floor and the shoulder blade in. Once they are over the head, observe the spaces between the elbows and the shoulders. If the elbows are locked or one side is lifted, fold a blanket horizontally and place it under the elbows.

What to do

Bring that shoulder blade in and continue to move the arm up and back. As you press the feet to the wall and extend the legs, move the shoulder blades in, lift the chest, and move both sides of the waist back toward the floor. Press on the side that is ungrounded and lift the side that collapses.

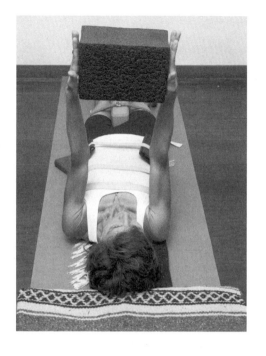

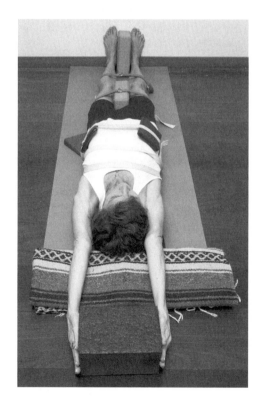

Variation 4: With Asymmetric Arms

Props

Three blocks, blankets, belts, small pads, wedges.

Benefits

This variation differentiates and lengthens both sides

Placement

From the previous variation the arms now will move toward the upper diagonal while the legs are extended with the feet on the floor.

What to do

As you press both feet on the wall, press the hands on the block, lengthening and move the arms to the right. Try pressing more with the left foot to create a resistance.

If you have a right thoracic curve, bring the right ribs further in as the left side and ribs elongate.

If you have a lumbar curve, work from the feet and legs. Press the left foot and bring the left hump in toward the spine. Press both feet and elongate the lumbar spine. Return to the center and change sides. If the curve is on the left side and the lumbar curve is on the right, stay on this side longer.

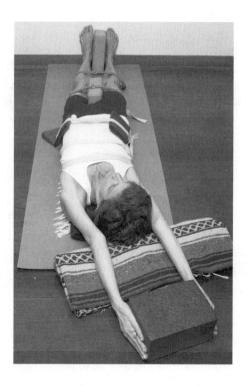

Variation 5: With Thumbs Hooked

Props

Mat, wall, three blocks, two blankets, two belts, wooden wedge.

Placement

From supta tadasana with feet on the wall, lift both arms up perpendicular to the shoulders, hook the right thumb with the left thumb, and extend both arms over the head. Bring the arms back in line with the shoulders and over the head. Change the hooking of the thumbs so that the right thumb is hooked over the left thumb.

Note

Use pads to support the shoulders, to lift the thoracic spine, and to fill the space for the concavities.

Benefits

Hooking the thumbs improves the asymmetries because it lengthens the side of the body, stabilizes the shoulder blades, and creates space for the chest to spread.

What to Do

Press the feet to the wall and extend and lower the legs as the thumbs hook. Both the extended arms and the shoulders move away from the ears. If the left side is the concave side, add an extra reach of the leg and pull from the left thumb, and move the left ribs up and to the side. The next action is to move the arms away from each other to move the shoulder blades in. This isometric action of the arms creates firmness and stabilization for the shoulders and for the chest.

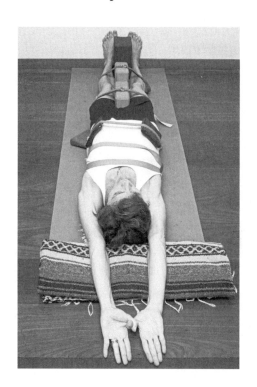

If the hooking of the thumbs is closing the chest, release it, align the arms with the shoulders, and open the hands with the palms facing the ceiling.

Both eyes look equally at the ceiling.

You can choose one of these variations, or do them all. When you are done, if there is time, do the following:

Remove all the props and just lie flat on the floor and map your body. Observe and compare from how you first lay down and after experiencing these variations.

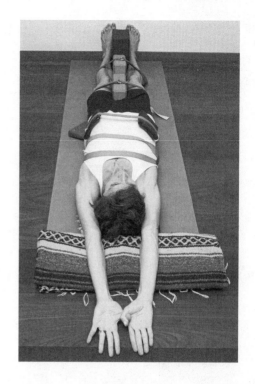

SUPINE VARIATIONS OF STANDING POSTURES

Supine Utthita Hasta Padasana: Lying on the Back with the Arms and Legs Spread

Props

Mat, wall, blankets, pads.

Benefits

The broadness of this position brings stability for both sides of the back and tones the arms, legs, back, and abdominal muscles.

Placement

Place the mat with one end by the wall. Fold a blanket in a vertical shape that will support both ends of the spine (the tailbone and the back of the head). Lie down on the middle of the mat and extend each leg down, moving into supta tadasana. Next, spread the legs about four feet apart and move your arms in line with the shoulders, palms facing up, unless suggested otherwise. To check the alignment of the limbs, look at each hand and make sure that they are both in line with the shoulders. Look at the feet and make sure that they are parallel and your toes are extended.

What to Do

Press the four corners of the feet on the wall, extend the legs, and press the thighs down. The top of the legs are securely rooted in the joint, and the outer hip turns inward. The tailbone reaches down and the pubic bone up. Both sides of the waist move back toward the floor. Roll the shoulders away from the ears and the outer shoulder blades in. Extend both arms until the back of the upper arms touch the floor. From the extension of the arms, roll the convex side of the rib cage inward and spread the concave side outward. Open the middle of the chest to the right and left sides. Release and return to supta tadasana.

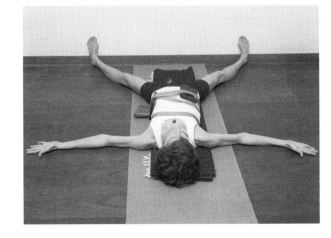

Variation 1

Turn the right leg out. If the left hip lifts, use a small pad under the right outer hip. Repeat on the left side.

Note

If the back moves away from the floor, increase the height of the blankets. Both sides of the back should feel supported.

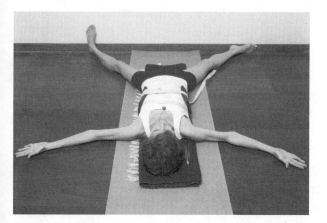 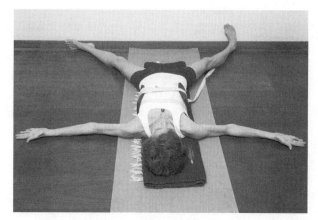

Supine Vrksasana: Tree Posture on the Floor

Props

Wall, mat, blankets, one block, two wooden wedges or pads.

Note

This lying down position can be done without the wall. However, it is best to do it near a wall so the feet can press against it and signal the rest of the body to lengthen.

Placement

Before lying down, arrange all the props near you. Fold one or more blankets to support the spine and the concavities. Make sure that the props are near you. Bend the legs and lie down. If lying down is uncomfortable, increase the height of the support or use more blankets.

Place both feet on the wall, and gradually extend both legs in supta tadasana. As you press the left foot into the wall and lengthen the left leg, bring the right leg up and place the right foot against the left upper groin. The inner groin releases toward the inner knee, and the outer knee lifts toward the outer hip. In this position, there is an external rotation of the right thigh as both hips compact inward (imagine two slices of bread coming together to form a sandwich). The anterior pelvic rotation from the scoliosis will be highlighted, as one hip lifts up toward the ceiling and the other rotates back toward the floor. Use wedges on the outer hip to bring the pelvic halves into alignment. The external rotation of the right thigh (the bent leg) will move the left lumbar curve to normal alignment.

What to do

Holding the outside edge of the block with the palm of the hands, slowly lift both arms up to a perpendicular angle, hands facing the ceiling, reestablishing the shoulder position as you move the upper arms down and the shoulder blades in, focusing on the shoulder of the convex side. Continue the action so both arms are over the head. Ideally, the arms are in line with the shoulders; depending on the degree of your curve, the proper alignment may not be possible. In this case, add extra props—a wooden plank under the chest or a folded blanket—to open the chest. If the arms cannot move back, fold

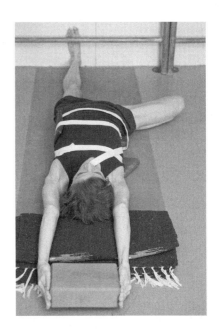

a blanket to provide support. If the elbows and wrists are lifted, fold the blankets and place them under the elbows and wrists for hyperextension.

The foundation of this asana is the standing leg. Reestablish the length as the left foot presses on the wall, especially if the left side is the retracted side. Move the left hip away from the rib as the foot presses, the arms lengthen overhead, and the right foot (bent leg) presses on the left groin. Both ribs lift away from the pelvis. The convex rib will be heavier; use a wedge or pad under it to promote a lift. The eyes look toward the ceiling.

Go back to supta tadasana and change legs. Use the wall as a floor and the foundation for this pose. Use an extra blanket for the back and concave spaces.

Left side

From supta tadasana, as you lengthen the right leg and press the foot on the wall, bring the left leg up, and place the right foot against the right upper groin, as the left groin releases toward the inner knee and the outer knee lifts toward the outer hip. The gravitational pull will help release the joints and the extra muscular holdings. Assuming that this is your contracted side, the action is to move the left leg out to create more space for the torso. Imagine someone pulling on the legs to release the tension.

Supine Ukatasana: Powerful Posture

Props

Mat, blocks, blankets, wooden wedge, pads.

Benefits

This posture strengthens the legs and induces midline orientation and compactness.

Placement

Fold one or more blankets lengthwise to support both sides of the whole spine, including the back of the head and the tailbone. Lie down and assume supta tadasana. Bend both legs and place the feet together with the soles on the floor near the buttocks, with the knees over the center of the shinbone and feet; if the knees are turning in, use a small pad or a block to support them. Hold a block with the palm of the hands and the fingers facing up. Lift the arms over the head. If you are unable to bring the arms back, fold one or more blankets or use a bolster to bring both arms back and to support the elbows. Observe the position of the tailbone, both sides of the lower back, the upper back, neck, and head. Note which side seems to move away or move toward the floor and make both sides even by performing the opposite action.

What to Do

As the feet press evenly on the ground, the outer shins hug in, the outer legs and hips compact in (without squeezing the thighs together) and stabilize toward the midline. As both hands hug the block, the shoulders roll back and away from the ears, the back spreads and the spine lengthens. Compact the convex ribs in and lift the middle of the chest. Ground the concave ribs from the front to the back as the ribs spread.

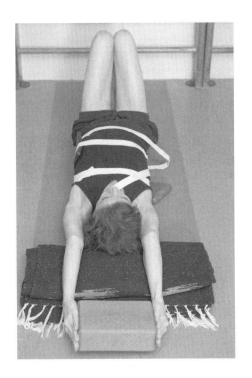

Note

If having the legs together causes discomfort and pain, change the position of the legs and decentralize the position. Spread the feet pelvis-width apart, with both feet parallel and both knees perpendicular to the feet.

Variation 1: Without the block

Repeat the exercise as if you were holding a block.

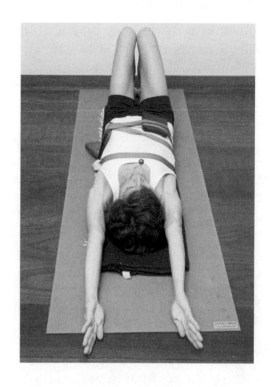

STABILIZING THE CORE FROM THE SIDES

Anantasana is a side-lying balance, and it establishes the side midline. It is a difficult posture for those of us with scoliosis. The following is a modification of the classic posture. It will improve the proprioception of the sides, enhance awareness of how to work with the various curves, and stabilize the front and back of the body while lying on this side line position.

Modified Anantasana: Vishnu's Coach

The principle is to lengthen and strengthen the concave side through the extension of the limbs and to restrain the convex protrusions with the support of the props. For lumbar scoliosis, fold a blanket or use the pads under the apex of the lumbar hump. The idea is to prevent the spine from collapsing.

Props

Wall, mat, bolster, three small blocks, blankets.

Benefits

This side-lying position increases core, pelvic, and shoulder stabilization, and also focuses the mind. The support of the block or blanket from underneath is used to have the convex ribs and lumbar hump gravitate to increase mobility on the less mobile vertebrae and to move the spine medially. The firmness of the block gives a clear proprioception of the bones and how to correct them. The wall gives support and proprioception to the back of the body and induces the front (abdominal organs and muscles) to rest toward the spine. In the first variation, the bolster is like a wall.

Placement

Ideally, you will need assistance for these variations because the setup requires refinement. Place a mat adjacent to a wall. Have a bolster on the center of the mat and in contact with the wall. Before lying down, place one flat block between the inner ankles, another one in the back of the buttocks, and a third in a place where the convex rib can lean against it. Lie down on your left side with the back to the bolster. Adjust the props or have an assistant help set them up. The feet are positioned together as in tadasana. The back touches the bolster without collapsing on it. Extend the left arm and rest the left ear on the upper arm. The right hand stabilizes on the floor at a right angle with fingers facing front. Once there is a sense of balance, extend the right arm on the side of the right leg with the hand facing down; the left arm is extended on the floor under the left ear. If the extension of both arms brings instability, place the right hand back on the floor at a right angle with fingers facing front.

What to Do

As you lie on your right side, extend the legs, hug the blocks, and stretch the feet. Extend the right arm and press the right hand, moving the right convex ribs in and away from the prop as the right side lengthens. The right side moves in as the concave ribs move up toward the ceiling. Press the left hand on the floor and move the concave ribs toward the ceiling and away from the floor. Eventually, extend the left arm down onto the leg.

Come out of the posture by removing the props. Lie on your left side if this is the concave side and has a lumbar curve. Further lengthen the leg on the side of the curve. For instance, if the curve is on the left side, extend the left leg away from the left arm. Add a small rolled blanket like a sushi roll under the hump where the vertebrae feel less mobile. The extra lift will constrain the curve from further moving out and create space for the ribs to spread. Extend the left arm away from the left foot and press the left hand, spreading the concave ribs toward the floor as the lumbar spine moves in. Press, extend, and move the convexities in. For the ventral convexity, move it back.

Note

The rolled blanket has to be adapted; some people will need a thin roll, others will need a thicker one.

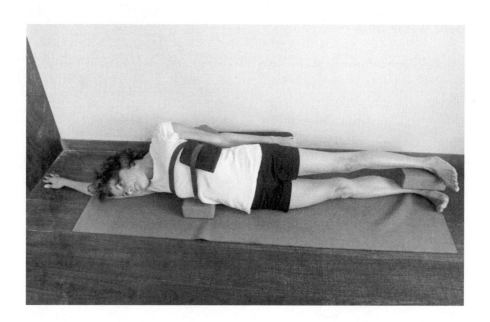

Variation 1: With Sandbag on Convex Ribs

Repeat the variation mentioned previously without the props, using the extension of both legs and arms to move the ribs accordingly. When lying with the convex side up, ask an assistant or a teacher to place a sandbag on the side of the convex ribs.

Placement

Lie on the side in the center of the mat with the feet touching the wall and with the concave side toward the floor. A teacher or an assistant will place a lightweight sandbag on the convex side ribs, in line with the apex of the curve, to induce the ribs to deflate and the spine to move medially. Crawl outward with the fingers until your arm is extended, palm facing down, and rest your head on your arm or a blanket if necessary. The opposite hand is resting on the floor or on the outer hip. Balance on the side. There is no need to place a weight on the concave ribs.

What to Do

Extend the legs and lengthen the arm. Compact the outer hips as the tailbone moves in and the pubic bone moves up. Lift both sides of the navel. Press both hands down and move the convex ribs in and move the concave ribs to the floor, extending the inner and outer edges of the legs firmly as in Tadasana. If you have a lumbar curve, press the lower leg further down and move the spine in.

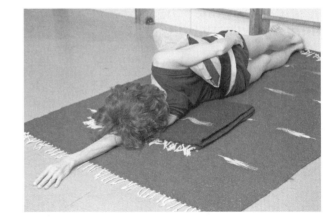

Lengthen both legs away from the upper body, and balance in this side-line position. Experience the sand bag constraining the bulges and inducing a compact side line balance.

PRONE POSTURE—LYING FACING DOWN

Benefits

Lying facing down is very soothing for the organic body, and most importantly, it is a position that releases and spreads the back muscles, allowing you to feel the back of your body. For scoliosis, this is an important position to bring awareness to the back with the underlying support of organic relaxation.

Props

Mat, blankets, pads.

Placement

Simply lie with the belly facing down and spread the arms and legs. If you feel that there is too much tension on the lumbar spine, fold a blanket and place it under the waist, use small pads to support the ventral convexities and concavities. Support the armpit with a folded blanket so the upper arms are in line with the shoulders, mainly on the protracted shoulder. You might also support the ankles with a blanket. Observe which side the head tends to face, and turn to the nonhabitual side. Observe which areas of the front of the trunk contact the floor and which do not, and use small pads to lift the concave areas that drop toward the floor. This means that the torso might need an extra lift. The upper arms are in line with the torso, and the forearms form a ninety degree angle. The palms of both hands rest on the floor.

In this prone position, feel your back, how the breath moves through both sides, and how it can fill and expand the concave side while pacifying the convex side.

Adho Mukha Virasana: Downward-Facing Hero's Posture

Note

Adho Mukha Virasana links the progression of lying to standing. It is a forward extension asana. It is important to have a teacher to learn this asana and how to modify it accordingly.

Props

Blankets, three blocks, weight, chair, wall.

Placement

Sit in on your heels with knees pelvis-width apart and toes touching in a position called virasana. Establish your sitting position by pressing both sitting bones onto the heels. Place one narrow vertical block under your forehead and one block under each hand. The height of the blankets and the position of the blocks will vary, but the blocks must all be of the same height. The final position of the buttock bones is grounded on the heels, and the forehead and hands are supported by the blocks. The head is leveled and aligned with the spine, and the arms are leveled and aligned with the shoulders for trunk extension. In this position, the concave areas should be supported with folded blankets. Fold an extra blanket and place it between the pelvis and the upper thigh approximately near the anterior superior iliac crest of the collapsed side. If the buttocks are lifted and thus not resting on the feet, fold the blankets so the pelvis is supported. If your knees and ankles hurt, fold a blanket on the mat and roll another one, not too bulky, and place it under the ankles. The rule for scoliosis is to support the concavities.

What to Do

Roll both buttocks down and press both sitting bones to the heels evenly as both arms and the torso extend forward. Press the right hand down and move the convex ribs in and down toward the floor. Extend the left hand out to lengthen and spread the concave left ribs.

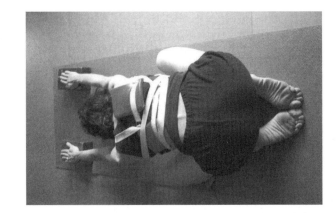

Press down with the buttocks as both arms extend up. Align the arms with the shoulders as you bend forward, and bring the head and the hands to the blocks to adho mukha virasana, press the hands on the blocks as the arms and trunk extend. Extend the arm of the concave side further as the buttock bone descends to the floor. Extend the arm of the convex side further. As the scapula moves in, the chest elongates. Press the convex side's hand down, and compact the bulging ribs in as the back side of the protruding ribs move down. The buttocks lower onto both heels. Move the collapsed areas by elongating the outer arm further and filling the areas from the front.

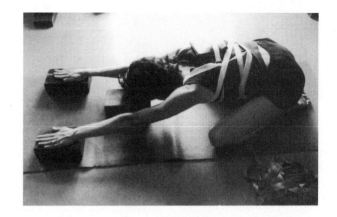

What to Observe

1. Notice the position of buttocks on the heels, the position of the big toes, and how they touch. In scoliosis, the big toe of the convex side will move forward. This reflects on the knees. Look at your knees, and observe if one knee is moving forward or retracting back. The knee that is moving forward results from the rotation of the pelvis and lumbar curve. Adjust from the feet, legs, and pelvis to the spine. Observe if both of the buttock bones carry the same amount of weight and which one is closer to the midline. Adjust by spreading the skin and muscles of the buttocks and then pressing both sitting bones down to the heel. The direction is to spread from the inside out to create space for the buttock and tailbone. Add an extra hands-on adjustment to open that buttock bone from inside out.
2. If your knees and heels are uncomfortable, roll a blanket and place it under the ankle joint and knees. Shift your weight to your feet. Fold extra blankets for the concave areas.
3. Notice which side of the trunk touches the thigh as the trunk moves forward and rests on both thighs. This is a place that will tell you how much support will be used to lift the concave side.
4. Notice the extension of the arms and the distance between the arms and the blocks as well as between the arms and the head. Observe the placement of both hands and both wrists. Are both hands and wrists anchored? Use the pressure of the hands to adjust both convave and convex sides.

5. The arm of the convex side tends to close the space between the neck and shoulders, and the front of the chest (the armpit) closes. To avoid closing the chest and lungs, de-centralize and extend the arms with the hands placed on the outer edge of the yoga mat. Do the same with the legs. If your knees and heels are uncomfortable, roll a blanket and place it under the ankle joint and knees. The weight shifts to the feet. Fold extra blankets for the concave areas.

6. To spread and elongate the lumbar spine, spread the legs so the knees are in line with the edge of the mat, with the big toes touching evenly. The convex ribs have to descend and the concave ribs have to lengthen in order for the convex ribs to compact toward the spine. The middle chest going down will move the convex torso toward the concave and open the space in the front of the chest. The concave side (flat side) has to find extra length from the left outer arm putting additional pressure of the hand. The ribs must be filled from the front to the back and move out.

7. When taking the arm and torso to the sides (asymmetric), finish the posture in the center (symmetric).

8. On breathing: The breath shapes and balances the concavities and convexities. As you breathe in, inflate the concave side from the front to the back. As you breathe out, deflate the convex toward gravity. Support the concavity of the right side created from the left lumbar scoliosis curve.

Variation 1: With Chin on the Block

Repeat the variation mentioned previously with the chin on the block instead of the forehead.

Benefits

The position of the chin induces the natural extension of the cervical spine and the elongation of the thoracic spine and chest, and with the help of the pressure of the hand it decreases the dome shape of the convex ribs.

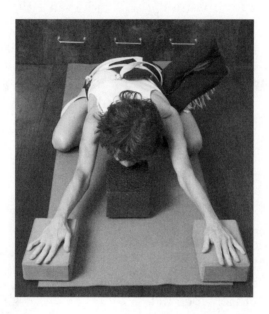

Variation 2: With a Chair

Props

Two mats, a chair, three blankets, pads, pranayama pillow, extra blankets to support the concave side, and a bolster.

Placement

Place the chair against a wall in the center of the mat. Fold a blanket and place it on the chair. Sit facing the chair in virasana. Support the knees and ankles if necessary. Do not have the chair too far away from you or it will induce a collapsed position; measure by the extension of both arms and hold the sides of the chair. The elbows are supported by the chair seat; if this is not possible, use a blanket. Roll as many blankets as necessary to support the torso; place as many folded blankets as necessary under the concave and collapsed areas, use a horizontal bolster to sit on if the sitting bones do not touch the heels; the principle is to support the concavities and fill the spaces. The knees are mat width apart. The big toes are touching, and the feet, in virasana, are extended—in particular, the little toes that hide as a result of the asymmetric spine.

What to Do

Extend both arms up as you roll the buttock bones down. Extend the inner and outer lines of the arms. As both shoulder blades wrap in, the sides of the trunk elongate and the waist moves back. Hold the back of the chair and rest the chin on the chair seat to lengthen the thoracic and cervical spine. Move the waist back to avoid arching the lumbar spine (hyper lordosis). In case of compression on the cervical vertebrae, move the chair closer and rest your forehead on it. The action of the chin will create extension for the front of the spine and space for the joints, discs, and ligaments. Pull the right hand down and move the convex side ribs in as the right side of the chest spreads. Pull the left hand and elbow out to spread the concave ribs and the scapula. Hold the back of the chair to extend both sides evenly, further stabilizing the convex shoulder blade that prolapses. Lastly, hold the elbows and rest the forehead to quiet the brain. It is important to stop tracking the asymmetries and just rest.

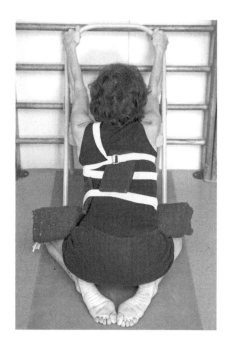

Variation 3: Parshva Adho Mukha Virasana—Lateral Reclined Downward Hero

In this variation, repeat the sequences with the arms moving to the diagonal; extending the arms and rooting the sitting bones will lengthen the opposite side.

Note

If the concave side is on the left, move both hands to the right and elongate both sides; add extra support for the left side if necessary. When going to the left, reach out rather than compressing; shift the convex ribs on the right side in and down. Stabilize both shoulder blades by bringing the outer edges of the blades in and lowering the tips away from the shoulders. Press harder with the left hand, and broaden the concave ribs to the side and toward the ceiling.

Props

Mat, blankets, blocks.

Benefits

For the proper benefits, the asymmetric spine has to move in all three dimensions. This will add mobility to the ribs and to the diaphragm, and will create a space between the intervertebral discs and vertebrae.

Placement

Repeat as for the primary Downward-Facing Hero variation. The suggested height for the block is medium height, to align the arms with the shoulders.

What to Do

Move the hands and the blocks to the right side to elongate the left side; use the breath in this side to further create motion between the ribs and the skin. The front of the body moves toward the back. Do not compress the concave side, allowing it to cave in further. The pelvis moves away from the ribs. As the hands elongate to the right side, the left buttock bone further descends to the prop. This creates a diagonal traction.

Return to the center.

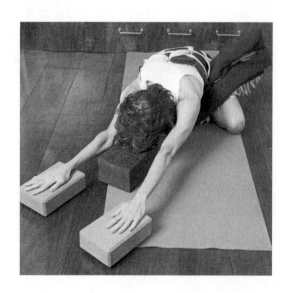

Left side: Move the blocks to the left as the right side elongates. If the left side is the concave side, extend the arms further out and increase the height of the outside block to further elongate and broaden the concave side. Simultaneously, press the right hand and move the right convex side ribs in as the front of the chest extends. As the arms further elongate toward the left, the right sitting bone grounds.

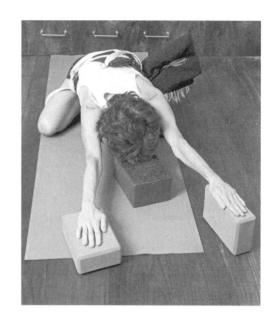

Caution

Do not push the torso down and further cave areas that are already collapsed. Instead, create space and fullness using the necessary props. Always go back to symmetry when doing asymmetric variations.

Note

The hand on the convex side presses down to move the side ribs in toward the center and down. The different block shapes allow the hands to act as a vector for elongation and create an imprint for the concave side to continue lengthening and broadening and for the convex ribs to compact in toward the spine.

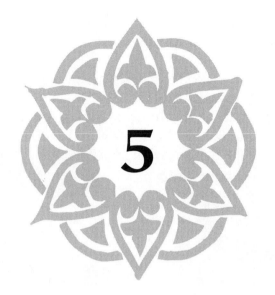

5

Standing Asanas

SUGGESTIONS FOR PRACTICING STANDING ASANAS

To view the traditional asanas, please refer to *Light on Yoga* by B. K. S. Iyengar.

1. Integrate the standing asanas into your daily practice. They will remove stiffness and pain and provide strength.
2. The use of props is necessary to achieve the best alignment and receive the healing benefits of the postures.
3. Compare how you feel before and after the yoga practice. Observe whether there is a feeling of space, height, energy, or harmony after practicing.
4. Observe how you stand on each leg and how your weight is distributed on both feet.
5. Feel the breath flow on both sides of the body.
6. In scoliosis, the ligaments and joints on one side are lax, and on the other side there is a pattern of hyperextension and tightness. Soften the joint and firm the muscles.

For instance, you can bend the knee slightly on the side that hyperextends and firm the tight muscles to lift the legs up. Make sure that neither knee is locked yet the thighs are extended and firm.

7. To improve focus and concentration, compact the muscles and keep the bones firm. An important attribute of the convex side of scoliosis (bulging ribs) is the way the skin envelops the muscles that compact the ribs in toward the spine. On the concave side, the ribs move away from the spine and touch the muscles and skin. Use the proprioception of your hands and touch to inform the mind of what adjustments need to be made to achieve symmetry of the ribs.

TADASANA

Mountain Posture

In tadasana, the extension of the legs begins from the distribution of weight of both feet. There are many receptors in the 26 bones, ligaments, and muscles of the feet. These inform the nervous system how to organize posture, align, and be present in life. The feet are part of the mature muscular skeleton; when misaligned, they will cause a deviation of the legs, pelvis, and spine, resulting in poor locomotion and perceptual problems. The feet are the foundation for a healthy posture.

Things to Observe

The weight between the right foot and left foot is uneven in scoliosis, so the feet require different adjustments. Observe which side bears more weight. Which knee tends to bend and hyperextend?

A practical way to adjust the knee that flexes is to press the foot and slightly shift the weight to the heel to extend the leg. Conversely, the concave side knee tends to hyperextend. Bring the weight slightly to the ball of that foot and extend the leg. In case of differences of leg length, a small pad under the heel will help to stabilize the joint and bring evenness.

For the classic postures, please see *Light on Yoga* by B. K. S. Iyengar.

Note

For the following variations, the feet may either be together or pelvis-width apart. When the feet are apart, the asymmetries are better accommodated, and the weight is more evenly distributed. If you are in pain, widen your stance further. When the feet are together, you will become more aware of your midline and increase your concentration and focus. This position also calls attention to the unevenness of the spine. The straps shown in the several photos are for a right thoracic curve; they help the stabilization of the shoulder blades and offer a compact feeling for the trunk. The straps reestablish the integral relationship of the skin, muscles, and bones, offering a solid feeling and sensitivity. Ask a teacher to help you find the best way for you to use the belts.

Variation 1: With Back Against the Wall

Props

Wall, mat.

Benefits

The wall provides feedback by allowing you to feel which parts touch it and which do not. This position is also good for strengthening the core.

Placement

Place the mat along the wall. Stand with your back touching the wall, with feet and legs together, and ankles and toes touching. Your arms are at your sides. Concentrate on pressing four parts of the foot into the ground: the big toe mound, the little toe mound, and the inner and outer heel. Observe the deviations and try to correct them. If one leg is longer than the other, place a pad under the heel of the short leg.

If bunions prevent you from bringing your feet together, either spread your heels or slightly separate your feet.

What to Do

Put your feet together, open and spread the feet and toes, stretch the sole, and adjust your weight by pressing the four corners of each foot into the ground. First, lift all the toes up and stretch the legs by lifting the muscles of your thighs. Then, relax your toes and maintain the extension of the legs from the feet to the spine. Move the thighbone back toward the wall and lengthen your tailbone toward the ground.

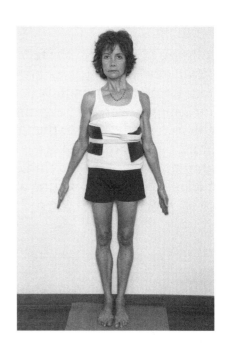

Note

If one of the legs is hyperextending, bring the weight to the ball of the foot, and soften the back of the knee.

As both legs extend evenly, the tailbone reaches down, the very bottom of the abdomen lifts up, and the waist moves back toward the wall. Don't be discouraged if one side of the back does not contact the wall. Address the correction from the front of the waist to the back. Relax the front of the ribs, and lift the back. Move the convex ribs and shoulder blade in and forward, and move the concave ribs toward the wall while spreading them to the side.

The areas that drop are activated from the feet to the spine. The thigh moves back and up, and both outer hips compact or firm in.

Move the back of the head, top of the shoulders, and back of the upper arms to the wall, and extend the arms evenly. Lower your shoulders, and move the outer shoulder blade in and down.

Learn how to adjust the proper space for the arms, because one arm moves closer to the body than the other. The sternum lifts as the chest skin spreads to the side, particularly on the convex side. Because of the protraction of the shoulder joint, the chest closes. To further open the chest, turn the palms of the hands to face the front of the room, and press the back of the hands on the wall.

Finally, keep your ears parallel as the back of the head moves back in line with the tailbone. Look forward evenly. Lengthen both sides of the neck. Align the center of the eyes, nose, and mouth with the center of the chest and navel and the center of the legs and feet.

Variation 2: With Legs Apart

Props

Mat, wall (optional).

Benefits

The widening of the legs is very important for scoliosis. As the base of support broadens, the weight is distributed evenly, accommodating asymmetries and creating a sense of stability and freedom. It also stretches the back and relieves pain.

Placement

Stand with the outside of your feet in line with the outer edge of the mat, and extend the arms next to the body.

What to Do

Press the four corners of the feet, roll the big toe mound down and lengthen the inner and outer edges. Lift the thighs up and back as the tailbone lengthens down and both sides of the waist move back. Extend both legs evenly and lift the ribs away from the hips by pressing your feet. Press the foot on the concave side and lift the ribs as you feel the convex ribs move in toward the spine. Extend both arms and reach with your fingers. As the shoulders move down and away from the ears, the shoulder blades move in.

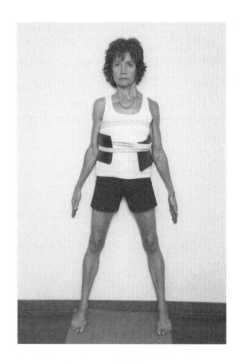

For shoulder stability, turn the palm of the hands to the front. Then, maintaining the firmness of the shoulders, turn the palms toward your body.

Repeat the actions of the first variation.

Variation 3: With a Block

Props

Mat, block.

Benefits

This posture orients the legs to midline.

Placement

Place a tall block vertically between your ankles. Observe the weight between both feet and which inner ankle tends to contact the block and which does not. Check whether the weight is distributed evenly between the balls of the feet and the heels.

What to Do

Press the four corners of the feet, lengthening the inner and outer edges. Move the inner part of your ankles away from the block and lift the knees toward the groin. Bring the upper thighs back as the tailbone reaches down and the waist moves back. Extend both arms and reach with your fingers. As the shoulders move down and away from the ears, the shoulder blades move in.

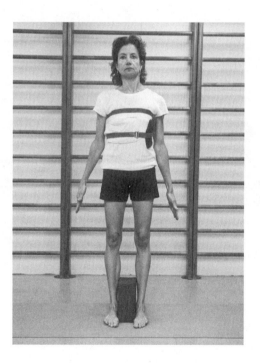

When the foot rolls, it indicates that the head of the femur is not centered in the joint, which is the result of lumbar asymmetry.

The extension of the legs will be from the inner ankle to the inner groin.

Repeat the actions of the first variation. Press, lengthen, and spread the soles of the feet, touch the block with the inner ankle, and extend the legs up from the inner heels to the inner groin as both outer hips firm in. Extend the arms up in Urdhva Hastasana (Upward Hands Pose), and roll the shoulders back as the outer shoulder blades draw in.

Variation 4: Arms in Urdhva Hastasana-Upward Hands Pose

The lifting of the arms creates a sideline extension and decompression on the ribcage. Breathing is improved, as the chest is lifting and broadening.

From variation 3, lift both arms up as you extend the legs. Move the convex side arm out to open the front of the chest as the concave side arm reaches up. Bring the outer shoulder blades in toward the ribs and gaze up from your chest.

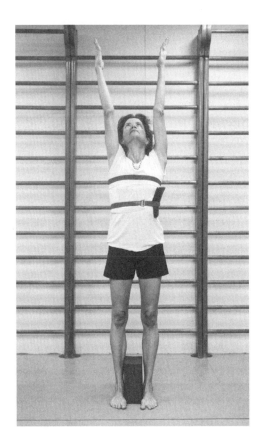

Variation 5: With a Plank

Props

Mat, plank or pole, broom.

Benefits

The wooden plank or pole helps the shoulders move back and away from the ears. As a form of external alignment, it provides stabilization for the shoulder blades, and a reference from which to adjust both of the sides.

Placement

Stand in tadasana and hold a wooden yoga plank, a pole, or a broom with your right hand. Spread the feet to the outer edges of the mat so they are parallel. Hold the plank from behind with both hands, palms up.

This posture may be performed with the feet together or apart in tadasana. Distribute the weight of the feet, extend the legs, relax the ribs in front, and lift those in the back. As you pull the plank down and roll the shoulders back, bring the outer shoulder blades in and down, away from the ears. Rotate the upper arms clockwise (from the inside out). Move the convex ribs in and spread the opposite side out. Lift the sides of the body up away from the pelvis as the sternum lifts and the chest spreads to the right and left sides.

Note

Press the foot of the concave side and lift the ribs, press down on the inner foot and big toe mound of the convex side, and move the ribs in.

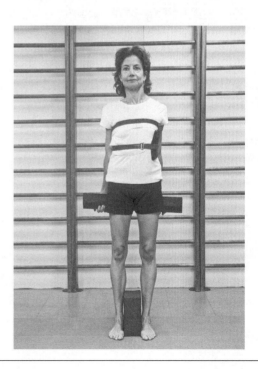

UTTHITA HASTA PADASANA: FULL EXTENSION OF ARMS AND LEGS

Props

Mat, wall, bolster.

Benefits

This stretch improves the extension of the limbs, allows proper distribution of weight, and provides proprioception as it tones the limbs and spine.

Placement

Stand in the middle of the mat in tadasana with your back to the wall. Spread the legs four feet apart; if you have no knee problems, jump into this position. This jump requires the arms and legs to be coordinated. At first, because the timing of legs and arms in scoliosis is not synchronous, the landing will be zigzagged. Work on coordinating the action to land symmetrically. The legs and arms should be fully extended in this position. The arms are in line with the shoulders, with the palms facing down unless suggested otherwise. To check the alignment of the limbs, look at each hand, and make sure it is in line with the shoulder. Look at your feet and make sure that they are parallel and that your weight is evenly distributed between them. The head and neck are aligned with the spine.

What to Do

From tadasana, spread the legs and arms. As you press the four corners of your feet into the ground, lift the muscles of your thighs up and back, reaching down with the tailbone and up with the pubic bone. As both sides of the trunk lift, the waist will move back toward the wall. Roll the shoulders away from the ears, and roll the outer shoulder blades in. Extend your arms in opposite directions, press the upper arms into the wall, and stretch your fingers. Simultaneously, move the outer shoulder blade in and lift the sternum. To come out of this position, walk or jump back to tadasana.

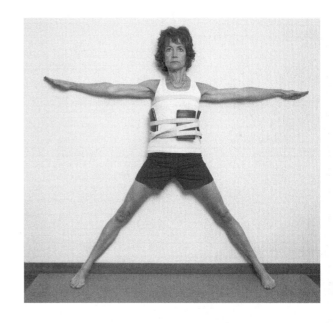

Note

If your back moves away from the wall because of the curve, place a vertical bolster behind you to support the whole spine, and adjust the position of your feet accordingly.

UTTHITA PARSVA HASTA PADASANA

This posture is similar to the previous one, but one leg is turned out. In standing asanas, one leg turns in slightly and the other leg turns out.

Props

Mat, wall, bolster.

Benefits

In addition to the benefits found in the previous exercise, this version addresses lumbar asymmetries, aligns and stabilizes the root of the leg on the hip joint, and tones, lengthens, and strengthens the legs.

Placement

Stand on the middle of the mat with the back to the wall in tadasana. Spread the legs to utthita hasta padasana, and turn the whole right leg out at a right angle. The middle of the thigh is in line with the knee, and the knee is in line with the center of the foot. Turn the left foot slightly in. Extend the arms in line with the shoulders. The back of the head touches the wall and is in line with the neck and spine. Fully extend your arms and legs.

Root the feet and extend the legs. As the whole right leg turns out to the side, rotate the back leg slightly in, press the back foot into the floor, and lift the thigh muscle up. Lift the pubic bone as both sides of the waist move backward. Lift both sides of the trunk from the extension of the arms.

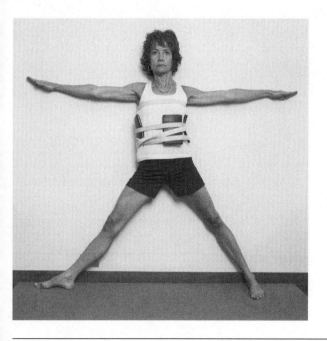 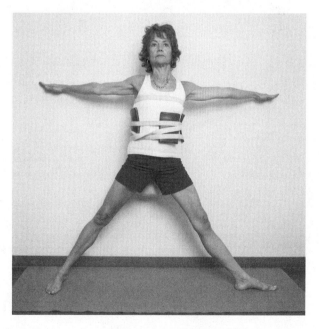

BALANCE, SPATIAL ORIENTATION, AND PROPRIOCEPTION

The vestibular system, located in the inner ears, is the primary center for equilibrium. These nerves sense the speed of movement, shifts of balance, and relationship to space, weight, and time through nerve cells called proprioceptors. These nerve cells or receptors are located in the joints, ligaments, muscles, and tendons. It has been shown that one of the causes of scoliosis can be the dysfunction of the vestibular nerves, affecting balance, spatial orientation, and an internal sense of the asymmetries. For instance, if you close your eyes the vestibular nerves will take over, registering your shift of weight, and directing your movement in space. They have their own vibration and wisdom. The yoga asanas in which the balance is on one leg, as well as the inversions, enhance the activity of these specific nerves even when there are imbalances. The eyes are related to balance, but secondary. For scoliosis, the asanas that address equilibrium are challenging, but they will teach you to rely on your inner ears and balance from the inside out.

VRIKSASANA: TREE POSE VRIKSASANA

Props

Mat, wall.

Variation 1: Standing Next to a Wall

Benefits

The practice of balancing on one leg—including teetering—with eyes closed will help to improve the equilibrium, stability, concentration, and self-confidence. This modified version of tree pose is very effective for scoliosis, and it forces the use of the inner ears. The wall is a reference to align the pelvis because the knee is fixed against it. The crawling of the fingers creates space for the rib cage and lengthens the external and internal costal fibers, which are important muscles for respiration.

Placement

Stand in tadasana with your left side to the wall. Bring the right foot to the left inner thigh, knee out to the side as the standing right leg lifts up like the trunk of a tree. Have the outside hand on the waist, and climb the wall with the inside hand (left). Once you have established your balance, lift both arms up with the hands facing each other. Come out by releasing in the reverse order, lowering the arms and then the leg.

What to Do

As the left knee contacts the wall, the sitting bone moves in line with the knee. Climb the wall with the fingers of your left hand, allowing your ribs to lift and spread. The right hand is on the waist as the right shoulder moves back and the right ribs move in.

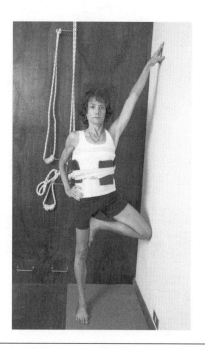

For a right thoracic or double curve, lift the right leg and externally rotate the right leg by moving the right sitting bone and groin in line with the right knee. Both hips compact and create pelvic stability as the pelvis opens and both sides of the trunk lengthen. For this side, use the action of the fingertips pressing on the wall to create stability for the shoulder joint and to move and compact the convex ribs toward the spine.

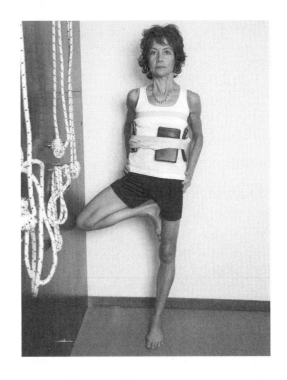

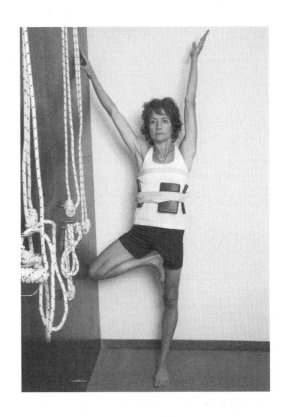

To learn how to balance independently, lift both arms up in urdhva hastasana with the palms facing each other. To come out, lower the leg and stay in tadasana.

To experience the proprioception created by the inner ear, close your eyes and balance without the wall. Observe which side of the body tends to shift. Use the hand on the wall and open your eyes if you need to reestablish balance.

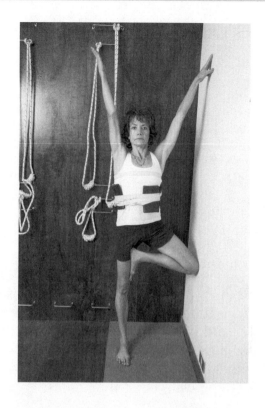

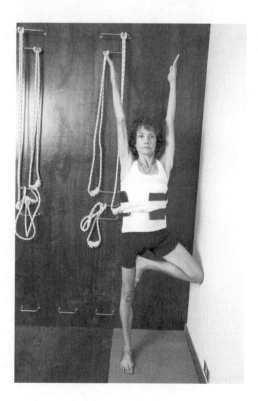

UTKATASANA: POWERFUL POSE

Variation 1: With Back to the Wall

Props

Mat, rope, wall with hooks for the ropes or exercise bars, belt.

Benefits

This posture tones the legs and core muscles (hip flexors, abdominal muscles), and increases symmetry.

Placement

Stand in the middle of the mat in tadasana, with the feet together or hip-width apart and the back touching the wall. Walk your feet a couple of inches out and bend the ankles, knees, and hip joints. The legs are at a right angle, with the knees over the ankles and in line with the second and third toes.

If the place where you practice has ropes, loop the long ropes on a high hook. With your back to the wall, bend the ankles, knees, and pelvic joints to enter utkatasana, and hold the upper ropes.

Observe how each side moves away from and toward the wall. On the convex side, the pelvis and shoulders rotate forward, whereas on the concave side, the ribs rotate forward. Use the wall as a reference as you even out these distortions.

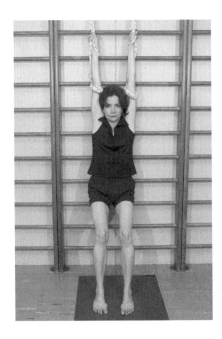

What to Do

Keeping your back to the wall, walk the feet out and bend the legs, reach the tailbone toward the heels, pull your pubic bone up and push your waist back to the wall (let the concave ribs press the wall and spread to the side, from the front to the back), and lift both sides of the navel up. Bring the back of the head and shoulders to the wall. As the legs move down, the sides of the trunk lift up. As the arms extend down, press the back of the hands on the wall, roll the shoulders back and away from the ears, compact the convex ribs in, and lengthen and spread the concave ribs out. To come out of the posture, straighten both legs and stand in tadasana. Repeat the exercise with the arms lifted up.

Note

If you have pain in your lower back, widen the feet to pelvis width.

The action of compacting the convex ribs comes from the skin moving to the muscles and the muscles moving the bone. The concave side is the opposite: the ribs expand the muscles to the skin.

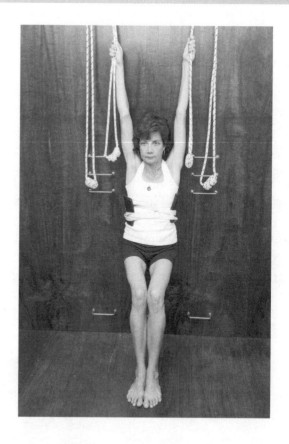

Variation 2: With a Chair

Benefits

This variation requires less strain on the legs and serves to improve your posture when sitting.

Placement

Sit on the front of the chair with feet and legs together, and lift both arms up with the hands facing each other. The upper arms are in line with the ears. The thighs, knees, and lower legs are centered over the middle of the feet (between the second and third toes). Observe whether one foot is moving forward and the other is moving backward; note the position of the knees and pelvis. Is one sitting bone receiving more weight? Are the upper arms in equal distance from the shoulders and ears? Move the arms apart (decentralize) to create space in the shoulders and chest.

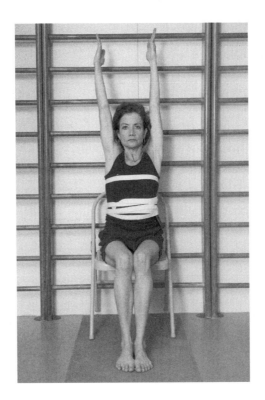

What to Do

Press down and spread the feet as in ta-dasana. Distribute your weight between the right and the left sitting bones, manually spread the flesh under the sitting bones, and root both sitting bones. Repeat this action twice to double-check the asymmetries. The outer hips firm in as the tailbone draws in and the pubic bone pulls up. The arms extend up, and the sides of the trunk lengthen. On the side that drops (concave), press the foot and extend the arm further up; lift the ribs away from the pelvis, and spread them to the side. Pressing the foot of the convex side, rotate the right pelvic bone back, moving the outer hip and the ribs in, and extending the arm as the outer shoulder blade moves in. Refine the posture: press both feet, root the sitting bones, and stabilize the shoulders by moving the arms away from the ears and drawing the shoulder blades in and down. Lift the chest bone up and spread the chest to the right and left sides.

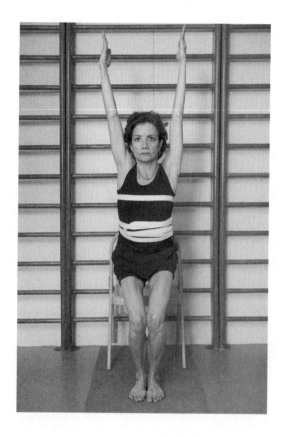

UTTHITA TRIKONASANA: EXTENDED TRIANGLE

Props

Wall, block, chair, mat, and block.

Note

The props in this exercise are designed to help you learn how best to align both sides. You can use a tall or flat block, or use a chair if you lack stability. It is important to experiment; your body will let you know which props work best for you. Note that the block position is different on each side. On the right side (convex), the block is in front of the foot for best alignment of the arm and shoulder blade; on the concave side, the block is further out to elongate the concave ribs. The alignment of the legs is also different for each side.

For a lumbar curve, the leg must be angular, with the heel in line with the toes of the opposite foot.

Benefits

This posture strengthens the legs, stabilizes the hip joints, and elongates and improves both sides of the rib cage (convex and concave). The rotational component of the torso works with the counter rotation of the spine.

Placement

Right Thoracic Convexity

From utthita hasta parsva padasana extend both sides of the torso toward the right as the left heel presses the floor. Place the right hand on the block that is in front of the right heel. The right shoulder blade moves in and the right ribs rotate toward the ceiling.

What to Do

Press the four corners of your feet. Lift both thighs up and firm the outer hips in. As you extend to the right, press the block to move the buttock bone in line with the heel, compact the right ribcage in toward the spine and slightly move the head to the back, in line with your coccyx. Extend the left arm up. Rotate the convex ribs toward the ceiling as the left heel and foot press back. Extend both sides and bring the waist back. Gaze up at your left hand or look to the front.

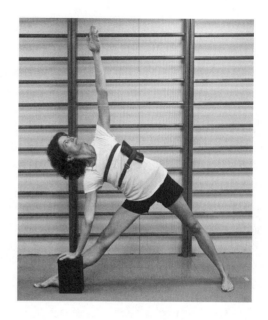

Left Side

Concave Side and Lumbar Curve

The block will now be further out to the side to elongate and concave ribs and side.

The left foot will move angularly forward. As the foot presses down, the left buttock moves in line with the left heel and the pelvis rotates toward the ceiling. Extend the right arm up in line with the right shoulder and bring the outer shoulder blade in. Maintaining the elongation of the trunk, gaze up or look to the front.

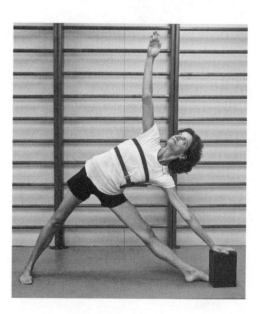

Variation 1: With a Chair

Placement for Right Thoracic/Left Lumbar Curves:

Stand in Tadasana with the back to the wall. Spread the legs four feet apart—your back is in contact with the wall. The feet are parallel, toes facing front. The arms extend to the sides and are in line with the shoulders (this is utthita hasta padasana). Rotate the entire right leg out from the root of the thigh. Your right heel should be in line with the arch of your left foot. Place a block underneath the ball of the right foot to bring the root of the leg into the joint; this is an important action for the convex side, because that side drops and the head of the femur loses its stability. Look at your right leg, and make sure that the middle of the thigh is over the center of the knee, and that the knee is over the center of the tibia and the center of the foot. If the major curve is right thoracic, the turning of the leg is important. Place the right hand on the back of a chair, next to the right foot. Lift up the left arm. As I am wearing specific straps for my curve, I use the left hand to pull the strap and the shoulder blade that protracts in.

Left side

Notice the different ways to modify both sides. For the left side I am using two blocks— under the ball of the foot to stabilize the head of the femur, and under the middle of the lower leg to inhibit hyperextension of the leg on the concave side. The strap is pulled in the opposite action from the concave side: it is pulled forward to bring the shoulder blade away from the spine.

What to Do

Right side

Press the ball of the foot on the block and press down on the outer edge of the left foot. Lift both thighs up and lift the sides of the trunk away from the legs as the right arm extends. Place your right hand on the chair, and lengthen the sides. Bring the right buttock in line with the heel, extend the left arm up, pull the strap with the left hand to move the right shoulder blade in, and use the right hand on the chair as a lever to move the right ribs in (bulging ribs). Move the head back in line with the tailbone. Look at the left thumb from the right convex rib. To come out of the posture: firm the legs, straighten the trunk, and face your feet forward in uttitha hasta padasana.

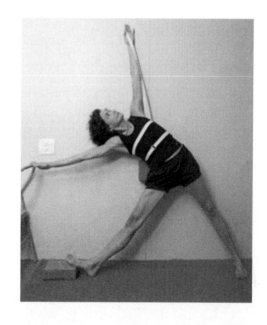

Left side

Press down on the ball of the foot and lift the thigh up. Move the left buttock in line with the heel, and move the trunk away from the legs. As the left arm extends to the sides and the hand holds the back of the chair, hold the strap with the right hand and move the left shoulder blade away from the spine—the right arm extends toward the ceiling. For the concave side, move the chair further out as the concave ribs lengthen. Extend the left arm and gaze at the hand maintaining the right convex ribs in.

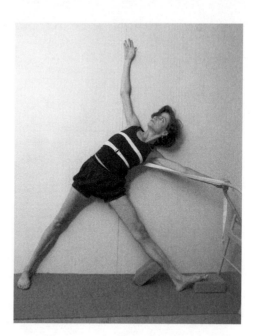

Note

Do not use use straps unless indicated by your teacher.

Variation 2: With a Looped Belt

Props

Wall, mat, 10-inch belt, two blocks or a chair.

Benefits

This variation increases the mobility of the hip joint, and when done in an angular stance it can further benefit the lumbar and double curves of scoliosis. Increasing the height for the front foot improves stability for the hip joint. The angular legs will affect the lumbar spine and its asymmetries, because the legs are the conduit for lumbar elongation and derotation. Address thoracic curves using props.

Placement

Have two blocks and a chair closer to the right side of the mat. Stand on the middle of the mat next to the wall in tadasana. Spread your legs four feet apart, (utthita hasta padasana), adjust the outer (left) foot so that it touches the wall. Turn the entire right leg out. Make a loop with the belt, and place one end under the arch of your left foot and the end with the buckle on top of the right thigh. Move the right leg to the front of the mat (slightly angular), and place the ball of the foot on a rolled mat or block. Extend the legs and arms in line with the shoulders, and from the hip, extend the trunk as you move to the right side. The right hand can be placed on the shinbone, on a block behind the foot, or on a chair. Do not rest your weight on the prop, but use the prop to stabilize the shoulder joint.

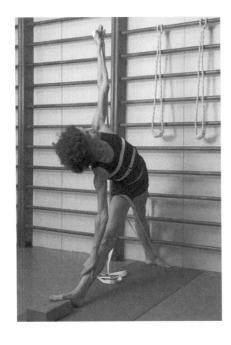

What to Do

Press the back of the left foot on the wall, and lift the thigh up to move the right buttock bone as the right leg further rotates out and the head moves back. Extend the arms, and reach out with the right arm, placing the hand on your shin, a block, or the back of a chair. Bring the right shoulder blade in and compact the right rib. Lift the left arm up toward the ceiling and extend the fingers. Rotate the head, neck, and trunk, and gaze from your right eye to the left hand. To come up, press the back foot on the wall, firm the legs, and lift the trunk to a vertical position. Bring both feet parallel, loosen and remove the belt, and return to tadasana.

Note

If the rotation of the head brings tension in the neck, maintain the gaze to the front.

The spinal belt, as seen in the photo, is to be placed under the supervision of a qualified teacher. In the photo, it is around the thoracic spine to offer stability to the shoulder blades and ribs—mainly the convex ribs that protrude out. In this variation, the hand is holding the end of the belt to extend the arm up and to induce the convex ribs and protracted shoulder blade to move in. This is not to be repeated on the concave side.

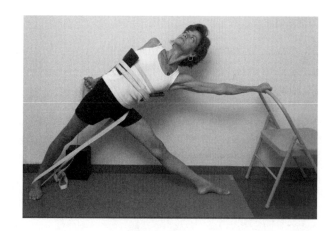

On the Left Side

Repeat the placement of the loop leg belt. Move the left leg to the front and the right leg slightly back to make the position angular. Press the back foot on the wall, lift the thigh, firm the legs, and elongate both sides of the trunk as the left arm reaches toward the left side. If the left side is the short side, it is important to use a chair or a tall block to elongate the concave ribs away from the hip. Extend the right arm up, and move the outer shoulder blade in as both sides of the chest spread. If you are using a spinal belt, do not pull it, but move the ribs to the belt. For the short side, we want the ribs to spread out.

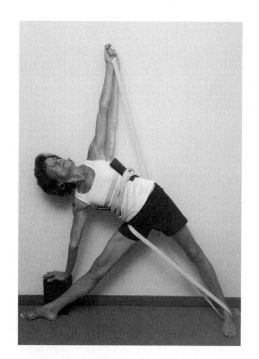

Note

For scoliosis, each side requires different placement of support. Once we understand how the sides need to move in a pose, we can use the same principle for all the asanas.

Variation 3: With a Rope

Props

Mat, wall, rope, chair, block or round wedge, long belt.

Benefits

Having the looped belt around the legs provides mobility for the hips and helps the lumbar spine elongate. Placing the front foot on a round wedge or block aligns and firms the head of the femur on the hip joint and enhances the action for the rotation of the thigh. Finally, holding the rope stabilizes the shoulder blade and allows the ribs to elongate and rotate.

Placement

Fasten a rope or belt over a window or on a hook high on the wall. Place the mat along the wall, and the chair or block by the right side of the mat.

From tadasana, move your feet four feet apart, keeping them parallel to each other. The outer edge of the left foot should touch the wall. Turn the right leg out: the right heel is in line with the arch of the left foot; the middle of the thigh is aligned with the knee, shinbone, and middle of the foot; and the knee is centered over the third toe. Place the ball of the right foot onto a rolled mat, a block, or a round wedge: the right heel is in line with the right sitting bone.

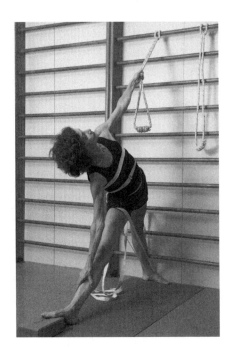

Press the left foot against the wall, lift the thigh muscle, and extend both legs as both sides of the trunk elongate to the right. Extend the right arm and place the right hand on the shinbone, a block, or the back of a chair. Move the outer shoulder blade in, compact the right ribs in toward the spine, roll the shoulders down, and spread both sides of the chest. Extend the left arm and hold the rope or belt. The rope is in line with the shoulder. Pull the rope, extend the arm, move the shoulder blade under, and spread both sides of the chest. Rotate the head, neck, and trunk, and look to the right hand. To come up, press the back foot to the wall, firm both legs, and lift the trunk up. Bring both feet parallel and return to tadasana.

Option

Use a chair, instead of the block, to improve the elongation of the ribs. If you are using a thoracic spinal belt, take the tail of the belt and lift it to help the convex ribs come in.

Left Side

If the left side is concave (right thoracolumbar scoliosis), the chair can be placed farther out. For a left lumbar curve, angle the left leg toward the front of the mat, according to your alignment; the principle is to have the inner and outer knee centered and over the foot, and the center of the left buttock bone moving inward so the lumbar curve is restrained. Work with the principle of the concave ribs spreading toward the skin and moving away from the hip.

Spread the legs four feet apart with the right heel touching the wall, and turn the left leg out. The sitting bone should be in line with the heel. Press the feet into the floor and lift the thigh muscles as the left hip moves away from the ribs. Elongate the left side, extend the left arm out, and hold the back of the chair. Extend your right arm and hold the rope or belt. Bring the right shoulder blade in and down. Keep your gaze forward.

To come out of the asana, press the feet into the ground, lift up, and lower the arm. Turn the legs parallel, and return to tadasana.

VIRABHADRASANA II: WARRIOR II

Props

Mat, wall, trestler, chair, bolster, blocks.

Placement

Stand in tadasana. Spread the legs five feet apart (wider than utthita trikonasana). Spread the arms to the side at shoulder level. Turn the left leg slightly in and the right leg out at 90 degrees. Look at the knee (perpendicular to the ankle joint) and align it over the center of the foot.

What to Do

Bend your right knee in a right angle, and press the outer edge of the left foot down. The right inner leg moves toward the inner knee, the outer leg moves toward the back side of the thigh. Both legs work in opposition to create space in the abdominal and pelvic organs. The knee is perpendicular to the shin, knee, and the space between the second and third toes.

The right arm and hand extend from the right lung and heart, whereas the left arm and hand extend from the left lung and heart. As both arms extend, roll the palms up to the ceiling as the upper arms rotate and the outer shoulder blades move in. Rotate your upper arms, but turn your palms back toward the ground. Be mindful of the pelvis, which tends to rotate forward on the convex side.

Turn your head to look at the middle finger of your forward (right) arm as the back arm resists in an opposing action. This position brings a relationship to the back and spine: the head is aligned with the tailbone. Extend the bent leg, bring the feet parallel, and return to tadasana.

Variation 1: On a Chair with Asymmetric Arms

Benefits

The variation on the chair places less strain on the muscles, and provides support for the pelvic floor from which both sides of the torso can lift in a vertical extension. The extension of the arms allows the torso to spread horizontally. The spine is kept stable. The wrapping of one arm and the lift of the other elongates the short (concave) side, stabilizes the shoulder blade, and opens the lungs as the arm folds in and back.

Props

Two mats, chair, wall rope, physioball.

Placement

Place your mat next to a wall, and center the chair on it. Use another mat as a cushion for the seat, and add a folded blanket to further increase the height if you are tall. Straddle the chair facing the back, bend your front leg and stretch out your back leg with the heel touching the wall. Instead of having both arms in line with the shoulders, lift the arm of the concave side up (as in urdhva hastasana), and wrap the opposite arm behind you. Gaze forward.

After learning to lift the concave side from the arm, do the asana symmetrically with both arms extended to the side.

For a right thoracic curve, wrap the right arm down as the left arm lifts up in line with the shoulder, with the palm of the hand facing in. If the convex side is on the left and the right side is the short side, lift the right arm up.

Note

You can repeat this arm modification in the first variation, but it is important to finish with both arms extended to the sides so that your body can learn how to integrate both sides evenly.

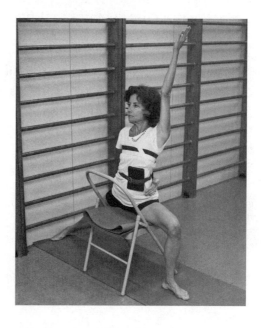

UTTHITA PARSVAKONASANA: EXTENDED SIDE ANGLE

Props

Wall, mat, block, bolster, chair, trestler.

Benefits

This is an excellent asana for scoliosis because the rib cage laterally flexes, extends, and rotates. For each side, the props, alignment of the legs, and hands differ. After learning how to work with both sides, integrate them.

Placement for Right Side

Place a chair and a block on the right side of the mat. Stand in the middle of the mat in tadasana, and then walk the legs four to five feet apart. Turn the left foot in, with the knee facing front. Rotate the right leg to a 90-degree angle, with the knee aligned with the center of the right foot. Bend the right knee to a right angle, and place a chair on the front side of the right thigh; rest your right forearm on the seat. This will offer a vector for the right rib cage (convex) and chest to move in toward the spine and rotate toward the ceiling (left side). Next, extend the left arm over your ear, holding the back of the chair and moving your right hand to the block on the front side of the right foot. If you are unable to reach this position, stop at the previous step.

What to Do

Extend the back leg and ground the back heel as the right leg bends in a right angle. Place the right forearm on the seat of the chair, and compact the right ribs in. Bring the left arm over the left ear, and extend the left side from the back heel to the hand as you hold the back of the chair. Let go of the block with your right hand and rotate the ribs up so that you can gaze at your left hand with your right eye. Now, move the left arm over the head and hold the back of the chair.

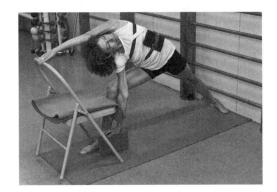

Placement for the Left Side

The chair position is different on this side and we are not using the block. Move the chair further to the left side so that you can lengthen the retracted side and ribs. Press the outer edge of the back foot on the wall and lift the thigh muscle up. As both sides of the trunk extend to the left, bring the right hand on the top of the hip to bring the right shoulder blade in. From the outer back heel, extend the right arm over the left ear in line with the shoulder. Maintain the elongation of both sides, and spread the chest.

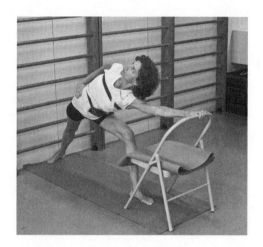 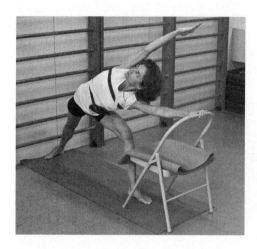

Variation 1: Seated on a Chair

Props

Mat, wall, chair.

Benefits

This exercise tones the pelvic floor from which both sides of the spine lengthen, the lumbar curve can feel gravity and decompress from the extension of the back leg, the rotational component of the ribs works with the thoracic curve and induce the proper alignment.

Placement

Place a mat next to a wall and a chair in the center of the mat. Straddle the chair with the right thigh on the chair and the left buttock bone off the chair. Press the back of the chair with your right side, and stretch your left arm over your head.

What to Do

Press down on the outer edge of the back foot, lift the thigh muscle, and extend the back leg. Move the right buttock in line with the right heel, and extend both sides of the trunk. Press the right hand on the back of the chair and rotate the ribs. Press down on the heel, and extend the left arm to elongate the ribs.

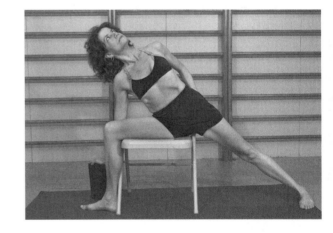

On the Left Side

If this is the concave side, to avoid patterns of collapse, modify the position of the left arm and place the left forearm on the thigh. Lengthen the left ribs away from the hips and stretch further to the side. You may keep your right hand on the back of the chair so your chest will move forward and your shoulder will move backward. The front leg is the fulcrum for the buttock bone to move in.

Variation 2: With a Bolster

Note

This variation is similar to the first variation seated in a chair, but adds a bolster.

Props

Mat, bolster, two blocks, chair, wall.

Benefits

The bolster constrains the convex side and induces the skin of the concave ribs to spread and move outward. The other props (chair, blocks) provide the proper height for the concave side to lengthen.

Placement

Perform utthita parsvakonasana on the right side. Place a bolster on the thigh and a block in front of the right foot. First, place your hand on your waist, and later, reach it toward the ceiling to create space for the upper left ribs and help the right curve move toward the spine.

What to Do

Press the back outer edge of the back leg into the floor, and move the right buttock bone in and under as the pelvis, chest, and head rotate to the left. Having the bolster between the torso and leg creates a resistance that counters the tendency of the convex ribs to gravitate. Lift the left arm as the left ribs expand out.

Concave Side

On the left side, add a chair for the left hand.

Note

In case of lumbar curve, the legs must be angled to achieve proper alignment of the hip and to bring the spine in.

Do parsvakonasana on the left side. Press the back foot down, and move the left buttock in. Rotate the pelvis and chest and lengthen the ribs. Reach with your left arm and hold the back of a chair. Reach your right arm up in line with your shoulder so that the shoulder blade wraps in. Relax your torso onto the bolster on your right thigh. For the concave side, release the tightness by moving toward the bolster. For the convex side, move away from the bolster.

ARDHA CHANDRASANA: HALF-MOON

Ardha chandrasana, like vrikshasana (tree pose), is a balancing asana. These exercises strengthen and reorganize the vestibular system, which is known to be weak in those with scoliosis.

Prop

Mat.

Benefits

With the proper support for each side, this asana offers a horizontal as well as vertical extension, helping to improve balance and proprioception as it strengthens the limbs and core.

Placement

From utthita trikonasana, bend the right knee, and place the right fingertips 12 inches in front of the right foot. Rotate the right leg as in trikonasana (external rotation). When the center of the weight is on the right leg, lift the left leg up until it is parallel to the floor as you straighten the right leg. Do not allow the leg to sag. Place the left hand on the lateral side of the left thigh to stabilize the shoulder blade, and lift the arm up.

What to Do

The tailbone tucks in as the lumbar spine lifts (front of the spine). Extend the limbs like starfish arms. Raise the back inner leg and heel, and straighten the right leg at the same time. As the left arm rests on your thigh, roll the shoulder back. Gaze upward with your right eye, and then extend the left arm. Avoid a banana shape. To come out, bend the right knee and go to utthita trikonasana.

Note

In any variation of this asana, be in a position to move the convex ribs toward the spine.

Variation 1: With Stools

Props

Mat, three tall stools, blocks, blankets.

Benefits

The support of the tall stools quiets the nervous system and teaches both sides to move in ways they are not accustomed to. It also offers a passive lateral extension, balancing both sides of the trunk.

Placement

Have three tall stools of the same height. A table or a counter might help. The principle is to support the back leg, the side of the torso, and the head. From utthita trikonasana, bend the right leg slightly, shift the weight to the right, and reach out with your right hand a few inches. Lift the back leg and support it with a padded stool or counter to align it with the outer hip. Adjust the right ribs on the second stool with a block for the right hand. Rest your head on the bolster and extend the left arm up in line with the shoulder. If you have a rope or wall with bars, hold the bar higher up with the left hand to move the left shoulder blade away from the spine and the ribs up toward the ceiling. If you don't have the extra prop, just reach the arm up toward the ceiling. Move the head back. Do not place your weight on the block.

On the left side, place the left ribs on the stool with a thin blanket on top. Use the left hand on a second stool or table to extend the left ribs (concave). Support the back foot on a stool or table. Reach up with your left arm.

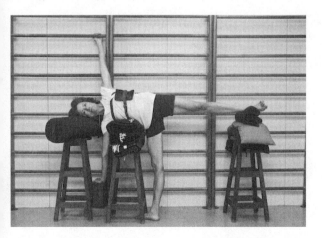 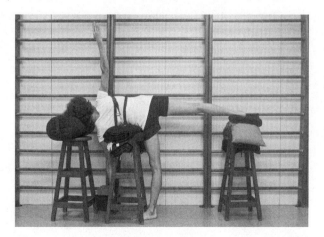

VIRABHADRASANA I: WARRIOR I

Prop

Mat.

Benefits

This pose is excellent for the eccentric contraction of the psoas major (the psoas major is a strong hip flexor that connects the lumbar spine to the thigh, and it has a major influence in lengthening and de-rotating the lumbar curve) because it opens the concave and retracted side, and offers release to the hip from the ribs.

Caution

All the standing asanas are very demanding, particularly this one. You should not perform these exercises if you have a heart condition. Primarily, be aware of the concave side of the scoliosis because this posture might aggravate it if performed incorrectly. Avoid the banana shape, which compresses the torso further. To perform this posture correctly, lift the lumbar spine, and move it back as the front of the spine lifts.

Placement

From tadasana, spread the legs four to five feet apart (utthita hasta padasana). Turn the left foot in 45 degrees, and the right foot out 90 degrees. Turn the trunk to the right. Adjust from the back foot so the hips face in the same direction as the right leg. Bend the right leg to a right angle. Place you hands on your waist. Make sure that you do not hyperextend your knee. Slowly lift both arms up, as in urdvha hastasana, and imagine that the chest has eyes that are watching your hands, especially from the convex side. Study the arm and hand positions; one arm will be closer to the ear than the other. Your arms should be in line with the torso and ears. Hold a block between your hands to improve the position of the arms.

Variation 1: At a Wall or Column

Props

Mat, wall, column, block, bolster, trestler, or counter.

Benefits

This variation tones and lengthens the inner legs. The bolster helps prevent the lumbar spine from moving forward, which is bad for any spine, but particularly for the spine in scoliosis that has a flat and compressed torso.

Placement

Follow the directions of the original posture but face a column or the corner of two adjacent walls. Place a bolster vertically between your body and the wall so the bolster will act as a column that supports the front of the body. Bend the right leg so the right groin touches the column. This position will help the right inner knee to move out. Lift both arms up in contact with the wall with the (convex ribs lifting away from the hips). Alternatively, lift the arm from the concave side up, and the arm in the convex side back. This action will lift the short side and bring the protruded ribs in.

What to Do

Extend the back leg as the tailbone draws in and the pubic bone lifts up. Raise the trunk, move the convex ribs in, and touch the bolster. Lengthen and spread the concave ribs; the outer shoulder blades slide in toward the ribs, the shoulders move down, and the chest bone lifts. As the arms reach up, the back heel extends toward the floor. Lift and extend the back leg and extend both sides of the trunk up. Release the arms, straighten the leg, and slowly come out of the asana.

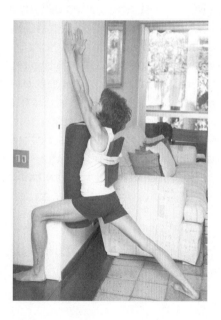

Note

Be aware of the concave side in this asana because the back tends to arch too much. The key is to bring the abdominal organs and muscles of the front body to support the back, from three actions: the tailbone drawing in, the pubic bone lifting, and the ribs moving away from the pelvis. The action for scoliosis is to lift the pelvic floor and both sides of the torso from the legs.

Variation 2: On a Chair

Props

Wall, chair or physioball.

Benefits

This posture tones and supports the pelvic floor, and lengthens the abdomen and both sides of the trunk.

Placement

Sit facing the back of the chair, thread the left leg in, and make a 90-degree angle. The heel of your back leg is on the wall. Hold the back of the chair and pull the arms in to lift the sides of the trunk. Next, lift both arms up, as in urdhva hastasana. Bend the right arm back as the left arm reaches. Come out in a reversed order.

What to Do

Press the right heel and extend the right leg back. Move the sitting bones down, and roll the right hip forward and the left hip back. If on a chair, hold the back of the chair and lift both sides of the ribs. Let go of the chair and lift both arms and lungs as the back heel moves to the wall. Lift the sides of the ribs—mainly the concave side—draw the tailbone in, and lift the pubic bone as both sides of the waist draw back. The kidneys move up as the tailbone draws in. Lift the pelvic floor, pubic bone, and lower abdomen up as the front of the spine extends. Come out in a reversed order.

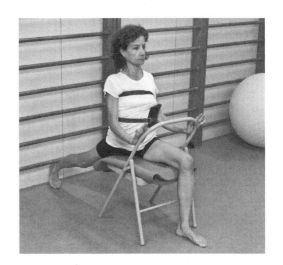

Repeat on the left side. If this is the concave side, keep the left arm up, and fill the concave ribs from the front to the back and away from the spine.

Note

The physioball is an excellent prop to strenghten the pelvic floor as well as balance. The bouncing of the ball offers spinal proprioception.

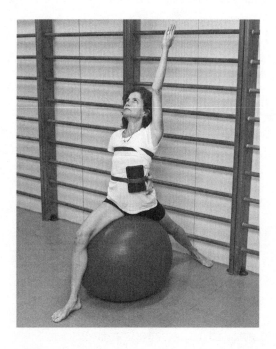

VIRABHADRASANA III: WARRIOR III

Prop

Mat.

Benefits

This asana, like vrikshasana, is about balance. This asana teaches you how to stabilize yourself by lifting up and aligning your center of gravity on the standing leg. For scoliosis—with the proper support—it tones the legs, the abdominal organs, and both sides of the trunk.

Placement

From tadasana, spread the legs to utthita hasta padasana. Bring your hands up to chest level, palms facing down. Lower your shoulders, and lift both arms up. Turn the left leg slightly in and the right leg out. Bend the right leg as in virabhadrasana I. Recline the torso onto the right thigh, shift the weight to the right leg, and simultaneously straighten the right leg and lift the left leg off the floor.

Variation 1: With a Chair

Props

Wall, mat, several blankets, chair, table.

Placement

Place a mat by the wall or counter and a chair with several blankets on it six to eight inches away from the wall. Stand in tadasana facing the back of the chair, and rest your upper thighs (root of the legs) against the blankets. Lean forward and place both hands on the chair seat for balance as you lift your back leg. Next, bring both arms up toward the wall in line with the shoulders. Use both hands to pull on ropes, a bar on the wall, a counter, or simply extend both arms. In this posture, the pelvis and waist are supported and so is the concave side.

What to Do

Stand in tadasana facing the back of the chair. Lean so that the back of the chair touches the top of the thighs, and your pelvis is supported by the blankets. Extend your back leg as the ribs move away from the pelvis. Extend your arms forward as your back leg reaches in the opposite direction. Lengthen both sides of the trunk through the extension of the arms, lift your sternum, and look to the front. Move the convex ribs toward the blanket and the concave ribs away and to the side. Reach from your chest and pull with your arms—pull harder on the concave side. Slowly, lower the back leg and come out of the asana.

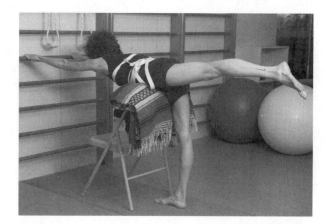

Variation 2: With Stools

Props

Mat, table, three stools, blankets, pads.

Note

The props are not set up the same for both sides. The convex side needs to move in and descend, so there is no need to place a pad underneath it. Conversely, the concave side needs to fill from the front to the back, so it requires support from underneath to prevent it from collapsing.

Benefits

This position stretches the entire spine, from head to tailbone, while supporting the front of the body.

Placement

Standing on the right leg, lean over a table or stool, making sure to keep both sides of the pelvis even. Lift the left foot back and onto a stool so that the leg is level with your pelvis. The height of the stool should be the same as the table; use blankets if necessary to make them equal. Flex your back foot, as in tadasana.

What to Do

Stand on the right leg, and lift the left leg back. Firm the standing leg and, as your torso rests on the support, lift your head up by extending your neck. Bring the convex ribs in and down toward the stool, and lengthen the short concave side by reaching forward with both arms.

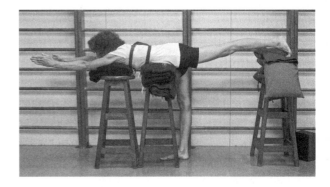

To do this exercise on the left side, stand on the left foot. If this is the concave side, fold a blanket under the left ribs. The height of the blanket depends on your individual needs.

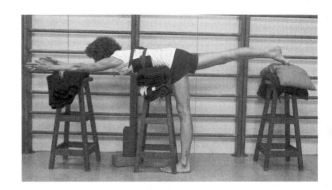

TWISTS AND SPINAL ROTATIONS

For safety and functional movement, your pelvis must rotate along with your spine, because the rotation comes from the soft tissue (organs). This coordinated movement is very important to avoid sacroiliac problems. Integrating the internal organs into the spinal rotation is vital in scoliosis, because the organic body provides the underlying support for the trunk, and therefore affects the asymmetry of the skeleton. On the short side, the organs are compressed and tend to adhere to each other. The twists are like oil that lubricates the organic structure through movement. The spinal rotation can be initiated from the pelvis to the chest and head, or from the head to the chest to the pelvis; the direction of the movement affects what your body learns from it. As the rotation gets fluid and deep, the bones and muscles stabilize as the organs slide, move, and find space. This is the mobility and stability of integrated movement.

A combination of standing lateral asanas and twists is the perfect way to work with scoliosis and its curves. In scoliosis, one side is retracted and lacks mobility, length, and strength. Although the convex side looks overly developed when viewed from the back, the anterior aspect of this side is concave, and the upper chest and armpit are retracted. Pay special attention to that side for length and space, and modify the asanas as needed. During rotation, the ribs and the lobes of the lungs move and broaden, so the breath can permeate the body.

To reach fluidity of movement in the organic body, repeat the rotation at least twice, and rapidly to both sides several times.

PARIVRTTA TRIKONASANA: ROTATED TRIANGLE

From this next session on, observe that the spine elongates from the extension of the legs, and that the legs act on the lumbar spine for rotation. The rotation of the thoracic spine stems from the action of the arms and the hands. Each side requires a different hand position and mechanical action, the specifics of which will be driven by you, based on your intuitive sense of your body. It is important to study and experiment with different pressures, pulls, placements of the limbs, heights, and props. The guiding principle is to create space and fullness in the concave (short) side, and to restrain the convex side as both sides elongate. Elongation is gained from opposing actions. The ribs move away from the hips, and the head reaches in the opposite direction from the coccyx. As one hand pulls, the other hand presses. The muscles of the convex ribs draw in toward the bone and spine. As the muscles of the concave side act in the opposing direction, they lengthen and move away from the spine toward the skin. The floating ribs broaden and lift away from the pelvis.

Props

Mat, block.

Benefits

This group of asanas works with the tridimensional scoliotic spine. They tone the legs and spinal muscles, provide organic mobility and circulation, and relieve minor back pain. In the latter stages of the practice they work with the derotation of the curves.

Placement

Stand in tadasana, and spread the legs three to four feet apart. Raise your arms out to the side at shoulder level (utthita hasta padasana). Turn the left foot slightly in, and from the root of the leg (hip joint), rotate the leg. Place a block on the inside of your right foot.

Rotate the right leg out 90 degrees from the hip so that you are facing to the right with both hips. Lengthen the spine forward, and place your left hand on the block. At the end of the posture, the hand is on the outside. Put your right arm on your waist. Twist the chest to the right, and extend your right arm out in line with the shoulder.

What to Do

Press the four corners of the feet down, extend both legs, lift the thigh muscles up and back, and tighten your hips in as both sides of the trunk elongate and rotate to the right. Place the left hand on a block on the inner edge of the right foot, and your right hand on your waist. Move the protruding ribs and the outer shoulder blades in as you lower your shoulders. Lengthen both sides of the trunk, and extend the right arm. Come out in the reversed order.

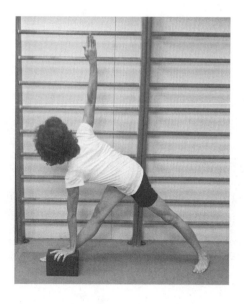

To the Left

The left leg is in front and the right is in back. Follow the previous procedure and, if this is the short side, as you twist to the left, touch the instep of your left foot with your right hand. For a right thoracic and left lumbar curve, use the block as on the other side. As you rotate, extend the legs and lengthen the left ribs away from the hip. Let the ribs stretch and spread.

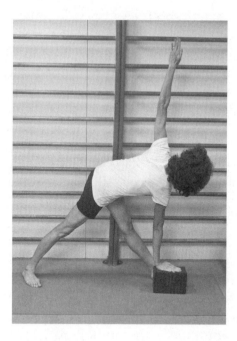

Variation 1: With a Block

Props

Mat, chair or tall block.

Benefits

The tall block or chair makes the posture easier and provides better alignment.

Placement

From tadasana, spread the legs four feet apart. Turn the left leg in at a 45-degree angle and the right leg out so that the outside of the foot is in line with the outer hip. Rotate to the right, and have the right hand on the hip. Place the left hand at an angle on the chair or block to open the retracted shoulder blade on the concave side, and to stabilize the left shoulder as the ribs and spine rotate.

What To Do

As you extend both legs back, lengthen the concave side, lift the ribs away from the hips, and extend the left arm as you place the left hand on the chair. Press the right hand and extend the arm in line with the shoulder as the legs continue to move back. If this is your convex side (right thoracic curve), from the extension of the right arm, bring the shoulder blade in and place it on the ribs to restrain the right ribs from moving back. Do not twist toward this side as you will be increasing the thoracic right curve instead of stabilizing it. Compact the spine as the belly softens and the navel revolves. Experiment with having the right hand up while looking at your foot, bringing the right ribs in and twisting from your belly. Gaze at your right hand with your left eye.

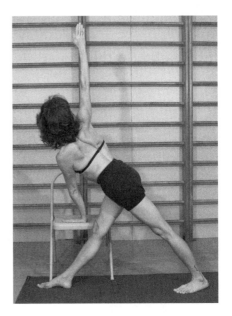

Left side

For this side, move the left leg forward and the right leg back. The right hand will now be on the chair.

If this is the concave side, extend both legs and move them back, pressing the right hand on the chair and lengthening both sides of the waist. Compact the convex ribs in as the left ribs elongate. Extend the left arm up and reach for the ceiling with your left fingers as the left ribs broaden. Gaze at your left hand from your left eye.

Variation 2: On the wall

Props

Mat, wall, chair.

Benefits

Improves proprioception, balance, extension, and the ability to counter-rotate the curves.

Placement

For this variation, the width of the legs and arms will vary depending on your curves. Stand with the back to the wall. Step the right leg forward and place the left heel on the wall. The back leg turns in, the right turns out, and the body faces the right. Lift the right foot up and place a block under the ball of the foot. If this is the convex side, the lift will bring the leg to the joint and provide better extension. The trunk rotates to the right and the left hand is placed on a chair to the outside of the right foot. The right arm extends in line with the shoulders.

What to do

Extend the legs and bring the outer hips in. As the spine elongates, pull the back arm and rotate the ribs. Firm both arms and lengthen the concave ribs away from the legs as the convex ribs move in toward the spine.

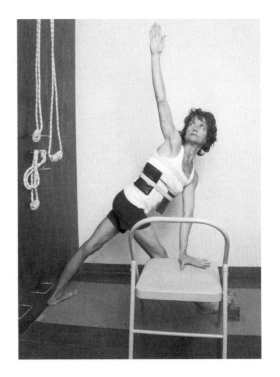

On the Left Side

Place the chair next to the left foot. Reach out to the seat with your right hand, keeping your left hand on your waist. Pressing with the right hand on the chair, move the right ribs in and elongate the left ribs as you extend the left arm up in line with the shoulder. The modified arm position (on the wall) on this side helps the concave ribs and side to broaden and lengthen. Place your right hand on the chair seat and extend your left arm up in line with the left shoulder. Reach for the ceiling with your fingers.

Press the feet and extend and move the legs back. Use your right hand as a fulcrum to rotate the ribs toward the left side. Extend both legs, compact both hips, and continue twisting to the right from the lower abdomen. The left eye looks up.

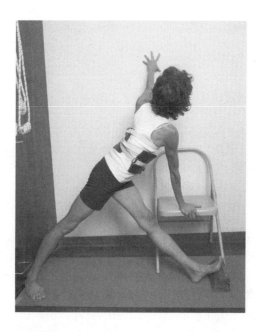

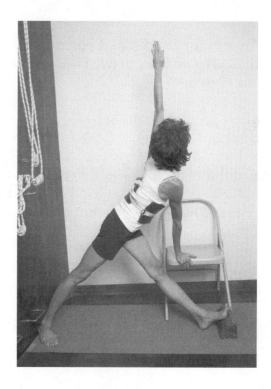

Variation 3: With a Chair

Props

Mat, chair.

Benefits

This decentralized position helps the fibers of the back muscles release away from the spine. The slight bending of the leg joints helps the center of weight to drop to the legs. The pelvis, ribs, and chest rotate. For minor pain and spasm, widen your stance.

Placement

From tadasana, spread the legs and arms (utthita hasta padasana). Bend your legs slightly, and twist to the right. Place your right hand on a chair seat and your left hand on your waist. Rotate the torso to the right from the movement of the floating ribs and kidneys. Extend both legs, compact both hips, and continue twisting to the right from the lower abdominal organs (liver, kidneys, and lungs). The left eye looks up.

Note

The liver is a powerful and voluminous organ. In a right thoracic curve, it is displaced to the right. The additional twist from this organ can enhance the space and movement of the convex ribs.

On the Left Side

Place the chair in front of the left foot. Reach out to the seat with your right hand, keeping your left hand on your waist. Press with the right hand, move the right ribs in, and elongate the left, as you extend the left arm up and then, as in utthita parsvakonasana, over the left ear. The modified arm position helps the concave ribs and side to broaden and lengthen.

PARIVRTTA PARSVAKONASANA: ROTATED SIDE ANGLE

Props

Wall, mat, two blocks.

Benefits

The blocks prevent the convex ribs from protruding. This variation provides a deep twist as it tones the legs, abdominal organs, and spine. The bolster brings more resistance and resilience to the side ribs.

Placement

Stand with the right side next to the wall. Bend the right leg, place a round wedge or a block under the ball of the right foot, and extend the left leg. Place a block between the ribs on your right side and the wall, and have another block for the right hand.

What to Do

Extend your back leg, stretch your head away from the left foot, and bring the convex ribs in as the left ribs rotate to the right. Note that for right thoracic scoliosis, stretch the head away from the back foot, extend the spine as the head moves away from the tailbone, and rotate the pelvis, chest, and head.

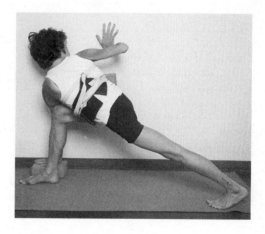

Variation 1: With a Bolster

Instead of a block, place a bolster next to the side ribs. As the trunk rotates, move the convex ribs in and the concave ribs toward the bolster.

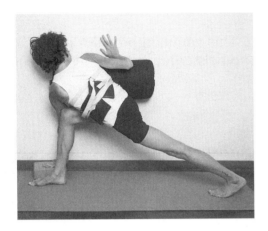 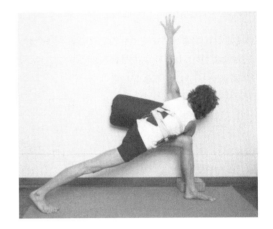

PARIVRTTA ARDHA CHANDRASANA: ROTATED HALF-MOON

Props

Mat, trestler or counter, stools, blankets, block.

Placement

Stand with the right side next to the trestler, counter, or table. Raise your left leg, and place your left foot on a stool, toes tucked under. Recline the torso on a second stool with a folded blanket under the concave side. Twist the torso to the right, and place the right hand on the top beam of the trestler or on the counter and the left hand on a block or stool; if this is not possible, have the left hand under the beam bar and the right hand on the top. Place a folded blanket under the concave side. Ideally, a third stool supports the back of the head.

To the Left Side

Place the right hand on a tall block and twist it back to lengthen and rotate the left ribs. If the curve on the left side is of the lumbar spine, focus on the derotation from the lumbar spine toward the right side, and stabilize the right shoulder blade and ribs.

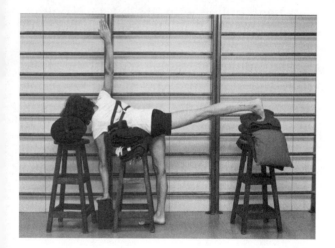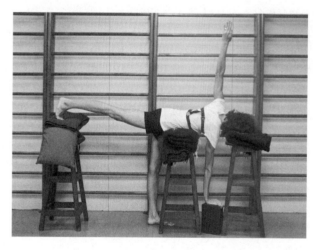

PARIGHASANA: GATE

Props

Mat, wall, blanket, blocks, chair.

Benefits

As in utthita parsvakonasana (side angle), parighasana has a lateral extension and a rotation of the spine: a perfect combination for scoliosis. It works directly with the lateral deviations and rotations.

Placement

Place a mat next to the wall, and fold a blanket in half. Kneel with the left side next to the wall, with the knees on the blanket. Bend the right leg at a 90-degree angle; the right heel is aligned with the right sitting bone and the left knee. Begin to climb the wall with the left hand and, if this is the concave side, move the ribs toward the wall but maintain the perpendicular angle of the left leg. Next, extend the right leg out to the side, and flex the foot (toes pointing up). Extend the right arm to the side in line with the shoulder, hand facing up. Extend the trunk to the right, as in utthita trikonasana and parsvakonasana, place your right hand on a block behind the leg, and put your left hand on your waist to provide stability for the shoulder. Extend your left arm over your head in line with the left ear. Look up first and then look underneath the left arm. Come out of the posture by bringing the right leg back to kneeling position. Repeat on the left side.

If the left side is the concave side, the convex ribs will be in contact with the wall; instead of moving them to the wall, do the opposite. The aim is to elongate the left ribs, even though the trunk is bending to the left, while compacting the convex ribs in. The degree of the lateral extension might be less on the concave side, but the important thing is to lengthen and compact the sides as you are able. The position of the block will change on each side. A chair can also be used to create height for the concave ribs to elongate.

What to Do

Extend both legs, move the thighs back, and twist from the inner body as the muscles of your back firm both sides. As you kneel, climb the wall with your hand, and lengthen both sides of the rib cage. Compact the outer hip in, move the root of the legs into the hip socket, and lift the pubic bone up and the tailbone in. As you place the right hand, roll the shoulders away from the ears and move the outer shoulder blade in. As the hand touches the block, move the convex ribs in and lengthen the concave side by reaching with the opposite arm over the head.

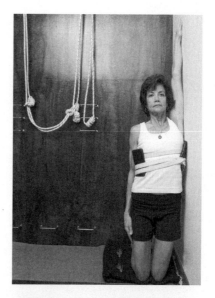

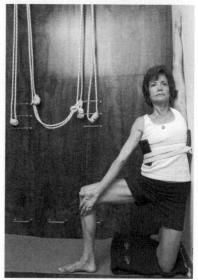

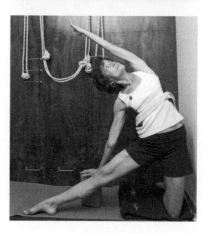

PARSVOTTANASANA: LATERAL EXTENSION

Props

Mat, wall, rope, chair, blocks.

Benefits

This asana tones the legs and spinal muscles, releases the tension of the shoulders, and lengthens the entire spine as the head moves away from the tailbone.

Placement

From tadasana, spread the legs three to four feet apart. Place your hands on your waist or clasped together behind your back. Turn the left foot in and the right leg out at a 90-degree angle. The torso faces right.

What to Do

Extend the legs, look up, and extend the torso forward. The torso lies on the right leg. The right hip is back as the torso moves forward. Bring your weight to the heel of your back foot. Release the back from the crown of the head as the torso continues to extend toward the front leg. Avoid rounding the back; maintain the tension between the head and the tailbone. Press the feet further and extend the legs. Create a full elongation of the front of the spine, with the head being the last to come up.

Variation 1: With a Rope

Props

Mat, wall, rope, blocks, chair.

Benefits

This exercise tones and strengthens the legs and back and lengthens the side body.

Placement

Stand with your back to the wall. Loop a wall rope around the root of the thighs (hip joint). Step the right leg forward, and place the left heel on the wall. The back leg turns in, the front leg turns out, and the body faces to the right. Lift the right foot up, and place a block under the ball of the foot; the lift will bring the leg to the joint and provide better extension. If you have a left lumbar curve, add a small block on the top of the right thigh, under the right waist, but not so high that it reaches the thoracic ribs. Place a chair in front of you.

What to Do

Press the feet into the ground and extend both legs, moving the thighs back as both hips compact—moving toward each other and providing the proper stability for the sides of the body to lengthen forward. Look up—not so much from the eyes, but from the middle of the chest. Extend the trunk forward in a concave angle until your hands touch the chair seat. Keep both hands under your shoulders as the shoulder blades hug the ribs. The middle of the chest on the convex side moves down, and the concave side moves back.

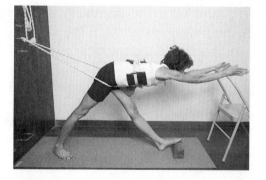

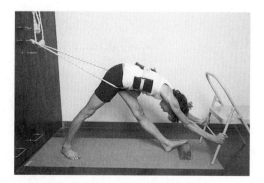

Move the hands out, rotate the upper arm, and move the shoulder blades in, especially the one on the convex side. The right lung lifts the right side of the rib cage, and the left lung lifts the left side. The sternum lifts as the chest opens. The lungs can now expand and fill on both sides—which is especially important for the concave side. Move the ribs away from the hips, again, focusing on the concave side. Note that the hand position in one is asymmetric to bring the protracted shoulder blade in.

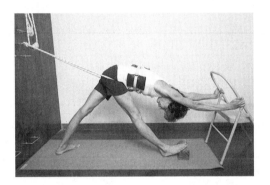

On the Left Side

Assuming this is the concave side, add an extra block to support the underside of the concavity—the front supports the back. Extend your legs, and bring your left hip back as the body extends forward from the hip joint—pause with the hands on the chair before extending further. Lift the side of the ribs, and then release the head.

PRASARITA PADOTTANASANA: WIDE-ANGLE LEGS EXTENSION

Props

Mat, wall, two blocks, chair, wooden boxes.

Benefits

In lumbar scoliosis, one sitting bone (ischium) moves back and the other rotates forward. The wall acts as a reference for the proper alignment. The ischial tuberosity (the two bony points of the buttocks) must touch the wall evenly.

Placement

In tadasana, with your back facing a wall, spread the legs five to six feet apart. The legs are parallel with the toes facing forward. Place your hands on your hips. Extend your torso forward from the pelvis. Place your hands on two blocks (the height will vary depending on your needs) directly below your shoulders. Both sitting bones touch the wall. Extend the arms and both sides of the trunk. Reach from your eyes and chest. Stay in this extension phase with the hands on a chair or blocks. The height can be gradually decreased if the alignment is maintained. Come up to position in the reverse order.

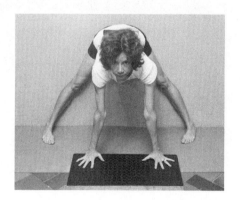
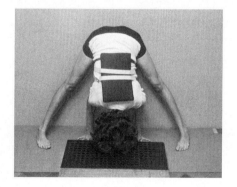

What to Do

Press the outer and inner edges of the feet, and ground the heels and mounds of the big and small toes. Extend the legs, and lift the root of the thighs as the sitting bones touch the wall and press into it. Lean your trunk forward from the pelvis, and place your hands in line with the shoulders on a block or chair—if possible, cup your fingers on the floor as the shoulders move back and away from the ears. Rotate the medial line of your arms out and the lateral line back. As the shoulders roll back and the outer shoulder blades move in, the middle of the chest moves in and the chest presses and lifts. Look up, continue the extension, and lay the crown of your head on the support. Your head should hang from the spine, and the lumbar spine (lower back) lengthens. Note that the extension is like in parsvottanasana from the front of the spine. Move the convex ribs in, and spread the concave ribs out. Both sides of the chest lengthen.

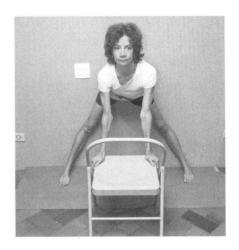

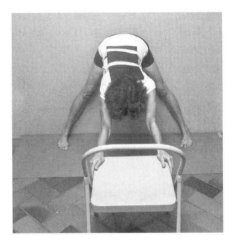

Note

Depending on the acuteness of the back's curve, it is very important to support both sides in the extension phase of the posture. Lean the trunk of your body on a platform or bench.

SUPPORTED UTTANASANA: SUPPORTED STANDING FORWARD EXTENSION

Props

Mat, high stool, two blankets.

Placement

Place one blanket over the stool, and fold a second one for the concave side. Place both feet outside the inner bar of the stool. Press the feet evenly and extend the legs. Lie over the seat, with the extra folded blanket under the concave side. Press the convex ribs down toward the stool as the concave front ribs move back. You may hold the legs of the stool as your torso lengthens.

What to Do

Move the convex ribs in toward the spine and the concave ribs away and toward the skin. Lengthen the front of the spine, and release the middle of the chest down. The inside of the legs should be perpendicular to the floor, with the sitting bones over the heels. The stool provides a passive extension; the back extends vertically and spreads horizontally.

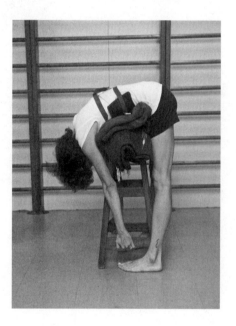

Variation: Supported Parsva Uttanasana-Lateral forward Extension

Repeat the variation above, but instead of facing the stool, move to the right side and extend and release the trunk.

This position offers the retracted side a chance to spread from the ribs to the skin. The intercostal muscles and their fibers begin to receive the nourishment of the breath, and the body can lengthen passively.

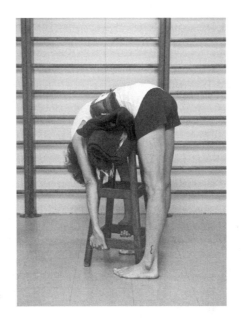

ARDHA UTTANASANA: HALF-FORWARD EXTENSION ON THE WALL

Props

Mat, wall, chair.

Benefits

This is a great asana to integrate in a daily sequence, because it trains you in stabilization of the shoulders, extension of the spine, and sideways mobility of the spine. On the apex of the scoliosis curves, the vertebrae lack mobility; they are difficult to move and to feel. The centralized and decentralized motion will add mobility.

Placement

In tadasana, face a wall and press the palms of both hands against it in line with the shoulders. Move your feet pelvis-width apart. Walk your feet backward and extend both sides of the trunk with the legs perpendicular to the floor, keeping your hands against the wall to indicate the relationship of the spine and tailbone, and how the line of force travels through the vertebrae. The legs are perpendicular to the floor. If your legs are hyperextended, bring your weight to the balls of your feet.

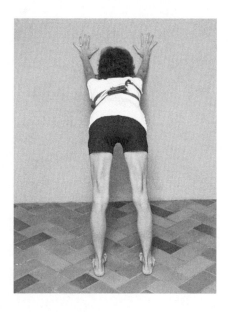

What to Do

Press into the ground and distribute your weight on your feet. Lift the thighs up and back, and move the sitting bones over the heels. Spread the hands and fingers, extend both arms, and lengthen both sides of the trunk. Press harder with the hand of the concave side, and move the ribs away from the hip. Make a convex shape on the back ribs. Press the convex hand and move the outer shoulder blade in and the shoulders down. Create a concave shape on the back ribs. Press and spread the hands, extend both arms, and lengthen the ribs away from the pelvis as both legs lift.

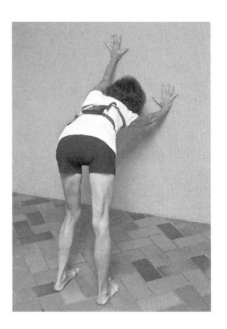

Note

For stiffness, add small lateral flexion (side bending), which will increase spinal lateral mobility.

Variation 1: With a Chair

Placement

Place the back of a chair on the wall. Stand in tadasana. Bring both hands to either side of the chair seat, slightly rotate your hands out, and walk backward, ending with your legs perpendicular to the floor, feet pelvis-width apart, and the sitting bones over the heels. Look up, and then lay the crown of your head on the seat; adjust your hands for better stability. Release and align the feet on the outer edge of the mat.

What to Do

Press the four corners of the feet into the floor, lengthen the inner and outer edges of the feet, and extend the legs by lifting the thighs. Extend both sides of the trunk and reach through the crown of the head. As you stretch the ribs away from the pelvis, move the convex ribs in and spread the concave ribs out. Further release the sides of the body and extend both legs. If you have a hamstring problem, add a lift under the heels. Walk back to the chair, and come up to tadasana.

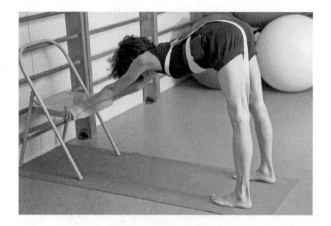

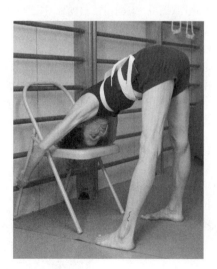

ADHO MUKHA SVANASANA: DOWNWARD-FACING DOG

Props

Blocks, chair.

Placement

From uttanasana, place your hands on blocks or a chair, and walk back. Start with the opposite leg than you usually do. Do not allow your torso to collapse; increase the height of the prop if it begins to do so.

The trunk action of adho mukha svanasana builds from adho mukha virasana. The middle of the chest, mainly the convex side, moves down or becomes concave, as the inner arm extends and the convex ribs compact in. Rotate your hands slightly to bring firmness and stability to the outer shoulder blades. The concave side arm extends more from the outer arm as the hand increases its pressure and the front ribs move back and spread to the side, creating a convexity on the back ribs. The diaphragm releases forward and the navel moves back toward the spine. This action is taken to the standing forward extension.

In cases of hip asymmetry caused from shortness of one leg, a small block can be used under the heel from the side that drops, or the side with the shorter leg. The same applies for the upper limbs; a small lift can be used under the wrist of the side that drops. For this exercise, it is particularly important to have a teacher to provide the proper support and help with the pelvic alignment.

For shoulder instability, elevate the hands on two blocks or a chair against the wall, and walk your feet backward. Not only will this help the shoulder alignment, but it will also remove the dead weight from the collapsed side and extend the legs back.

On the short or concave side, the bones and muscles move toward the skin. On the convex side, the skin and muscles move toward the bone. For the arms on the concave side, press the hand further as the arm lifts, the upper arm moves back, and the head of the bone stabilizes in the center of the joint. Move the hand slightly out to externally rotate the arm as the shoulder skin descends toward the lumbar spine. The concave ribs translate out toward the skin.

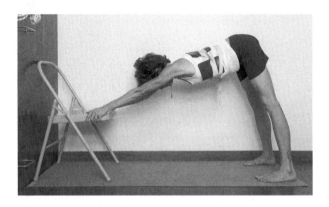

Variations

There are many variations of adho mukha svanasana. Here are some suggestions:

1. *With limbs spread away from midline.*
   Hands and feet are on the outer edges
   of the mat, stabilizing both sides. Add
   a support for the crown of the head
   (bolster, blankets) to calm and restore
   the brain. Place a support (bolster, blankets, blocks, etc.) under the chin bone
   to bring the convex vertebrae in. Widen
   your hands to increase the space between your shoulders and ears.

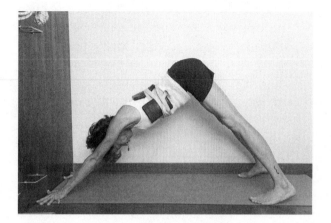

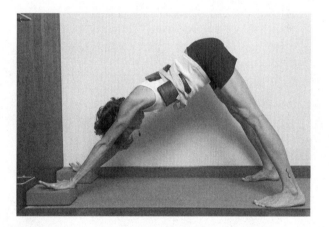

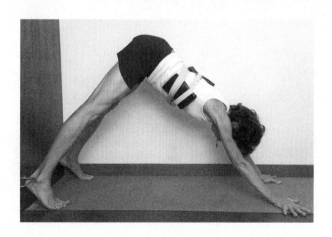

2. *Traction from ropes or belts.* Try it with crossed ropes on the wall and hands supported on blocks. The crossing can be with one rope or two separate ropes; the opposite leg will tread in the opposite loop. The crossed ropes provide a condition under which the inner legs lengthen as the thighs move back and the arms, the sides of the ribs, and the spine elongate.

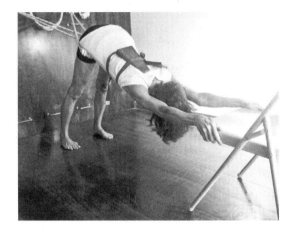

3. *Hanging from the rope and holding a chair.* This version further elongates the side body. Place the loop over the head and on the top of the hip joint; walk the feet back, and keep hold of the side of the chair. Lower your head and support it with a bolster. The lengthening of the spine comes from the extension of the limbs.

4. *Asymmetrical.* Repeat the previous step asymmetrically; move the chair to the right and elongate the left side. Then move the chair to the left and elongate the right side. To address lumbar deviation, stabilize the arms and move the legs to the side, emphasizing the length of the concave side and curve.

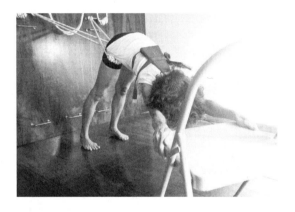

5. *Elevate the heels on the wall with blocks.* This will help to lengthen the hamstrings and legs and prevent the spine from rounding. A small lift under the heel of the side that drops can be very helpful for the leg to pelvis alignment.

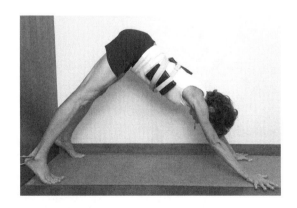

6. *Facing the wall.* Align your hands with your shoulders and your arms on two blocks, to lengthen the inner and outer arms and to stabilize the shoulder girdle as the middle of the chest moves in and spreads. Press your hands into the wall, pushing the root of the arm into the socket and moving the ribs away from the spine.

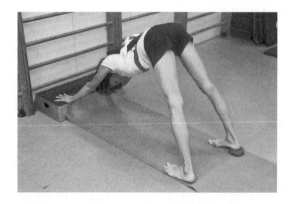

7. *Moving the hands and arms to the sides.* This asymmetric variation can be done with the ropes, a wall, a chair, or independently. When you move asymmetrically, always return to symmetry at the end of the exercise. This is an excellent version for scoliosis, because both sides of the torso can spread and move in and out as the spine extends.

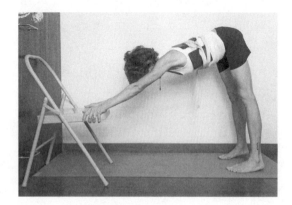

Place a mat along the wall and a chair on it. Face the chair with both hands down on the seat, and walk back to adho mukha. To do this asymmetrically, transfer the chair to the right side as the left heel moves down and the left ribs broaden. If the left side is the concave side, press down with the left hand, extend the arm, move the front ribs to the back, and create a convex shape on the back ribs. On the convex side, do the opposite: press the hand, extend the arm, and bring the shoulder blade and ribs in as the back ribs move in and down in a concave shape.

VASTISTHASANA: VASTISTHA-A SAGE

(Recommended for experienced students)

Props

Mat, wall, block, chair or physioball.

Benefits

This modified version for scoliosis strengthens and stabilizes the joints and central core. The spine has to balance between the front and back body. This is great for scoliosis, because the arm balance provides the action from which the ribs will compact and spread.

Note

The pad in the back gives proprioception of the back to protect the convexities and to bring sensation to the concavities.

Placement

From adho mukha svanasana, turn the body to the right side (as in anantasana). The balance will be on the hand and the outer edge of the right foot. The left hand rests on the left thigh.

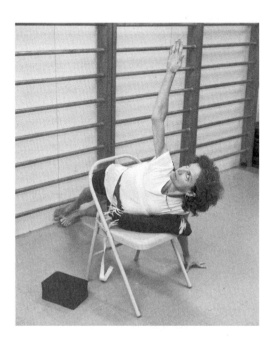

Variation 1: With Chair and Block

Props

Wall, mat, block, chair or physioball.

Placement

Sit near the wall and descend the side trunk on the chair. Have both feet next to the wall. Descend the trunk toward the floor as if you were going to slide, but instead, adjust the body so you will be lying on the side. Take a block and place it under the convex ribs. Extend the legs and have the feet to the wall. The right hand is placed on the floor or a block. The legs are parallel and the upper arm extends up in line with the shoulder. This is a sideline position.

What to Do

Extend the legs, compact both hips, lift the pubic bone up and the abdomen back. Roll the shoulders down and move the convex ribs toward the spine, and the concave ribs away from the hip and spine, as the head aligns with the tailbone.

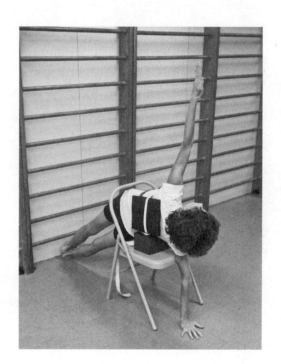

6

Seated Asanas

This chapter offers just a small modified selection of this very important asana group. To view the traditional asanas and their proper sequence and variations, please refer to *Light on Yoga* by B. K. S. Iyengar.

The seated asanas teach you how to sit with proper posture. The pelvis and the pelvic floor are the foundation for how you sit. Grounding and balancing your weight correctly on the pelvis allows the spine to rise correctly, resulting in an improved posture. In an asymmetric spine, this is not easy because the weight is shifted toward one side when the pelvis rotates. The teacher, the practice, and the props are the means to bring awareness of your natural posture and to create healthful ways to improve your alignment. The practice requires repetition, self-study, and assimilation.

SUGGESTIONS AND GUIDELINES FOR THE SEATED POSTURES

1. Before using any props, sit flat on the ground to learn your natural and habitual seated position. Observe and feel how the sitting bones contact with the floor, and whether one side drops or receives more weight. Note the position of your legs and your lower back.

   The height of the seat desired, with blankets, bolster, or chair, will vary from person to person. The goal is for the lumbar spine to be elongated, for the legs to be relaxed, and for the hip joint to be stable. A teacher can help you find the proper height.

2. Sit on the crown of the ischium (the bony protuberance on each side of your buttocks). Manually spread the skin and flesh of the sitting bones (ischia), and create a space on the pelvic floor. If one sitting bone moves closer to the midline, adjust again. Then, if one sitting bone is still receiving more weight, place a pad under the sitting bone on the opposite side.

3. Throughout the various postures, the term compact or firm will be used for the outer hip. This action comes from the contraction of the lateral hip rotators that causes the root of the legs (head of the femur) to move in the socket, which results in the stabilization of the hip joint and in the separation of the torso from the legs.

4. Use a support for the back, such as a wall, bolster, pillow, or block. Both sides of the back and the chest should feel lifted. Belts around the thoracic spine are helpful in relieving discomfort caused by the curve, and in bringing stabilization in the loose muscles and in the prolapsed shoulder blade.

5. The legs, when straight, should look like parallel tracks. Notice which leg tends to roll out and abduct (move to the side) and which leg tends to roll in and adduct (move in). Center and root the crowns of your heels. In tadasana (mountain pose), lengthen and spread the sole of the inner and the outer edges of the feet, including the toes.

6. If one leg is shorter or asymmetric, additional props (such as small pads) can be used to elevate the heel as well as the affected sitting bone.

7. Center the middle of your shinbone (tibia) over the middle of your feet (talus).

8. Lengthen the four corners of your knees by pulling the thigh muscles (quadriceps) and elongating the inner and outer ligaments. Observe the tendency of one knee to bend and the other knee to hyperextend. This tendency is often reproduced in standing, and the cause might be from the lumbar curve and pelvic rotation.

9. Align the middle of your knees with the middle of the shinbone, and approximately over the second and third toes of the feet.

10. In a single movement, root the middle of both thighs (femur) down, and move the head of the femur toward the hip socket (acetabulum).

11. To maintain the stability of the sacrum and the pelvis, you must lengthen the top of the sacrum bone nodes in the tailbone, widen the sitting bones, and lift the pubic bone.

12. Spread and move the lower ribs (floating ribs) away from the pelvis, especially on the side that drops (concave).

13. The diameter of the chest has to have the tridimensional space, mainly in the front and in the back dimension, because that is where the chest loses most of its space in scoliosis. Create a space between the chest bone (sternum) and the spine. Lift the chest bone from the bottom and spread the sides of your chest.

14. Move both shoulders away from your ears. The scapulae (shoulder blades), like two wings, are firm on the ribs, mainly on the convex side, where there is a protracted shoulder blade and less muscular support.

15. Press your fingertips down and back like an inverted cup to bring the shoulder blades (scapulae) in, to rotate the upper arm, and to lift the chest. The external rotation of the arm is an important action for the convex side.

16. Align your nose, mouth, middle of the chest, navel, and pubis. If you have a cervical or an upper thoracic curve, the head will tilt. Lift the ear on the side that drops, and keep your ears in parallel to bring the head to the center.

17. Each side of the scoliosis has to be treated differently. On the convex side, the ribs that protrude out, including those that provide an underlying support for the organs, must be compact and move toward the spine before lifting in the front. To create volume, lift and pull back the concave side or areas that cave in (flat)—the front ribs and the organic body. Spread the back ribs to the side. Lift the floating ribs (lower ribs) away from the hip.

18. Where there is a convex shape on one side, there is a concave shape on the other. Fill and push out the concave side to deflate and flatten the convex side. Support and elongate both sides as you search for evenness.

DANDASANA: STAFF POSE

While tadasana is the foundation for the standing asanas, dandasana is the foundation for the seated asanas. It is a symmetrical asana that provides training for postural tone and the symmetry of the legs, and it improves focus by bringing awareness in the midline and in the central nervous system.

Variation 1: Facing a Chair

Props

Wall, mat, chair, blankets.

Benefits

The chair serves as a support to adjust the asymmetries of the ribs and to lift both sides of the trunk. The extra height of the seat raises the lumbar spine and improves the posture.

Placement

Place your mat on the floor, with the short side against the wall, and put two to three folded blankets next to the wall. Set a chair in the center of the mat. Sit on the blankets with your back against the wall and face the chair. Stretch both legs forward, with the feet together under the chair. If your legs are hyperextending, fold a blanket under your knees but continue to stretch your legs and lower your knees. First, round your hands and place your fingertips on the floor with your hands next to your hips, thumbs facing forward and fingers facing back. Stretch out your legs evenly. Next, place both palms down on the chair seat and extend your arms in line with your shoulders.

Option

In cases of back pain or tightness in the hamstrings, spread your legs.

What to Do

Extend your legs, lengthen and spread the soles of both feet, press the crowns of the heels down, and pull the toes back. Stretch both sides of the knees and press the thighs down. While the outer hips are compact, lift the pubic bone up and pull the abdomen in. When both of the sitting bones are rooted and spread, the tailbone lengthens, the sacrum moves in, and your lumbar spine lifts. Press your hands on the chair seat, extend your elbows, and rotate the upper arm out and back, moving the outer shoulder blades in and up toward the ears. Using the pressure of both hands, compact the convex ribs in and lift and spread the concave ribs. Engage both sides of the trunk, spread the collar bones (clavicles), and lift your chest.

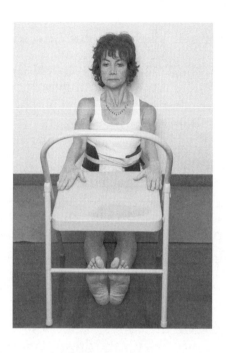

Variation 2

Sit without the wall, and spread your legs pelvis-width apart. Follow the directions mentioned previously.

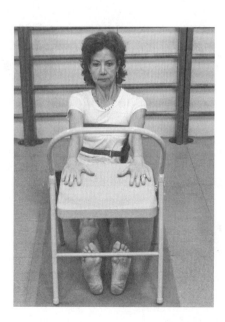

URDHVA HASTA DANDASANA: DANDASANA WITH THE ARMS UP

Variation 1: With Fingers Interlocked

With the arms up in urdhva hastasana, interlock the right thumb on the left thumb, with your arms in line with your shoulders and ears. If you are unable to sit in this position on your own, then sit against the wall. Change the hooked thumbs with the left thumb hooked over the right thumb.

What to Do

Using the actions from dandasana, extend both legs, firm the outer hips in, ground and spread the sitting bones, lengthen the sacrum, pull the tailbone down, and lift the pubic bone up as the abdomen moves back. With the arms lifted, hook the right thumb on the left and move the outer shoulder blade in. On the convex side, pull with the right thumb, extend the fingers and lift the inner line of both arms (medial line), as the outer shoulder blade moves in and down. On the concave side, change the hook of the thumbs. Pull with the left thumb, extend the fingers, and lift the ribs from the outer line of the arm as the left shoulder blade moves in and down and the concave ribs lift and spread away from the spine. With both legs extended and the sitting bones root down, lift the arms from the ribs and roll the shoulders back and down as the chest spreads.

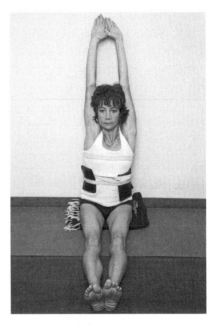

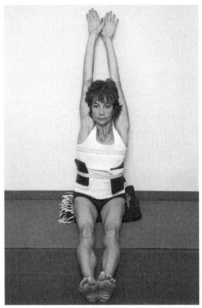

PADANGUSTHA DANDASANA: HOLDING THE TOES

Props

Mat, blankets, wall, belt.

Benefits

The extension phase of this posture is important for the health of the vertebrae. In scoliosis, there are many compressive and rotational forces acting on the spine. The extension of the spine with the support of the abdominal muscles can relieve back pain caused by these forces and improve breathing. In this posture, a belt or the thumb, index finger, and middle finger hold the big toe.

Placement

Extend your legs and fan and extend the toes up. Loop the belt on the right and left big toes and hold. If necessary, increase or decrease the length of the strap, but do not compromise the extension of the spine and trunk. Release and return to dandasana.

What to do

Extend and firm the legs toward the floor. As you press the ball of the feet the heels should press down onto the floor. Firm the outer hips in, and pull the strap evenly with both hands as the pubic bone lifts. Make the back, front, and sides of your body longer by extending the legs and pulling the strap. Lift the ribs away from the hips. Roll the shoulders back and down, away from the ears. Maintain contact between the shoulder blades and the ribs as the chest broadens.

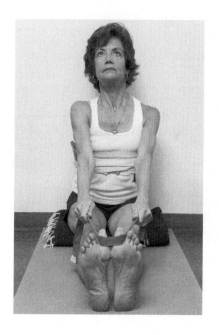

Fill the concave ribs by moving the front of the ribs to the back in a convex shape and by spreading the back concave ribs and skin away from the spine. Extend and press the legs down as the upper arms rotate out. Roll the top of the shoulders down, mainly on the convex side, as you lift, spread, and gaze up from your chest.

Note

Increase the height of your seat if the trunk is not extending. Do not round the back as this will cause harm to the vertebrae and spine.

Variation 1: Holding the Balls of the Feet with a Belt

Placement

Sit on one, two, or three folded blankets. Adjust and spread the sitting bones by moving the flesh and the skin away from the bone (repeat the action on the side that moves closer in). Loop a belt (six to eight inches) under the balls of the feet and hold it with both hands near the feet, as if holding the reins of a horse, so that both arms are extended. The spinal extension is activated by the traction between the feet and the hands.

What to Do

Extend your legs. Loop the belt and hold it. Fan and extend the toes up, and press the balls of the feet into the belt as the crowns of your heels move down. Firm the outer hips in and pull the strap evenly with both hands as the pubic bone lifts up and the abdomen moves back. Make the front, back, and sides of the trunk longer by lifting the ribs away from the hips. Roll the skin of the shoulders back and down, and move the outer shoulder blades in. Cave the convex ribs in by moving the center of the chest forward and by moving the outer shoulder blade and the side of the ribs toward the spine. Fill the concave ribs by moving the front of the ribs to the back in a convex shape and by spreading the back ribs away from the spine. Tense your legs, and rotate the upper arm out (the biceps and the deltoids move from the inside out). Roll the top of the shoulders down, lift and spread the chest, and gaze up.

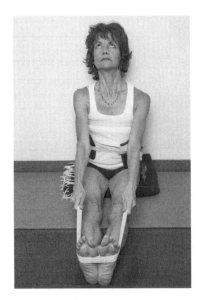

BADDHA KONASANA: BOUND ANGLE

Props

Wall, mat, chair.

Benefits

Helps to correct the placement of the ribs and to lengthen the trunk.

Placement

Sit on two folded blankets in dandasana, facing a chair. Bend each leg and move the knees to the side. Bring the heels closer to the groin, and put the soles of your feet together. Sit on the front portion of the sitting bones and lift the spine. The sacrum is lifted up and moved in. Place both hands next to your hips and lift the sides of the torso. Place the hands on the thighs to suggest a release. Interlock the hands and place them under your feet to lift the front of your body. Place both hands on the chair seat in line with the shoulders. The hands will offer the line of force from which the spine and both sides of the torso are lifted.

What to Do

Distribute your weight evenly, move the sitting bones apart, and spread the pelvic floor. Press the soles of your feet together and lower your thighs. The inner leg (inner groin) releases toward the inner knees, and the outer knees pull up toward the outer hip. As you press the chair with both hands, the pubic bone lifts, the abdomen moves back, the sacrum moves in, and the tailbone lowers. Lift the sides of the trunk, adjust the convex ribs toward the spine, and move the ribs of the concave side back. Lift the lower ribs away from the pelvis, and spread the upper back away from the spine.

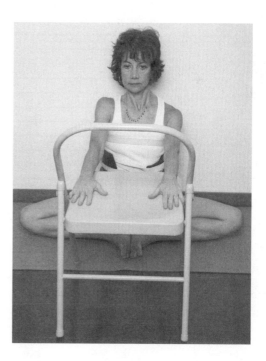

Note

If your postural muscles are weak or fatigued, sit with your back against the wall facing the chair. If your legs lift up, add another blanket to sit on.

Variation 1: To the Side

You can move the chair to the right to elongate the left ribs, and then return to the center position. Next, move the chair to the left and press the hands to stabilize the convex side. Taking the posture in a passive rotation is beneficial.

UPAVISTHA KONASANA: SEATED WIDE ANGLE

Props

Mat, chair, wall, blankets, blocks.

Benefits

This pose stimulates the flow of the blood in the pelvic organs, thereby enhancing their function. It extends the back, the inner sides of the legs, and the anterior and posterior sides of the spine.

Note

The pad under the heel is used to support the leg that collapses because of pelvic rotation. The height helps the leg ground in the socket and increases the extension of both sides of the knee.

Placement

Sit on one or two folded blankets in dandasana. Spread the legs to approximately 135 degrees apart, bring the weight to the front of the sitting bones, lift the spine, and extend both legs. Ground and spread the sitting bones apart. The right sitting bone is in line with the right heel and the left sitting bone with the left heel. Use the edge of the mat or the floor lines as references to check whether the heels are in line. Align your legs as in dandasana. Ground the crowns of the heels on the floor. Round your finger tips and face them toward the front with the thumb back. Move the hands slightly out to create a space for the ribs.

What to Do

Spread the feet, press the heels into the ground, and extend both legs by lowering the thighs and lengthening the inner leg (groin, knees, and heels). Pull your toes up and press the heels down, drawing the small toe and outer heel back toward the outer hip. Distribute your weight and spread both sitting bones. Lengthen the sacrum and the tailbone as the pubic bone lifts, the abdomen draws back, and the ribs move away from the hips. If the lumbar curve is on the

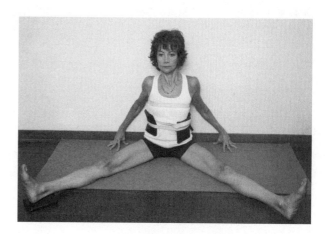

left side, extend the right leg from the inner groin to the inner heel, and gradually rotate the lumbar spine and the abdomen slightly to the right as the outer hips firm. If the curve is on the right side, extend the inner line of the left leg and slightly rotate the right lumbar and abdomen to the left. If your thighs lift up, press them down with both hands. Place the hands, rounded with fingers facing forward, on the sides of the hips. Check that the pressure of the fingertips is even, and lengthen the front, back, and sides of the trunk. If your convexity is on the right side, press the right fingers to bring the ribs in. If the concavity (short side) is on the left, move the left hand out to the side, press the fingers, and lift the left ribs away from the left hip and spread them to the side (away from the spine). Rotate the thumb out to bring the external rotation of the upper arm—mainly on the convex side. While the upper arm rotates outward, the outer shoulder blade moves in and down.

Note

The hands' position will affect the shoulders and the ribs. Widen the hands to the sides to create a space in the armpit, the chest, and the upper ribs, as well as to release the shoulders down. Press the fingertips and lift both sides of the trunk.

Variation 1: With a Bolster

Suggestion

In these variations, if one sitting bone is still receiving more weight after spreading, adjust them and place a pad under the opposite side and under the heel.

The variations focus on the extension phase of this asana that teaches the spine to extend from the front. The extension phase is the first stage that adjusts the asymmetries and relieves the compressions.

Note

Observe the alignment of the legs and the feet. The right and left heels should be in line. Lumbar curve asymmetries result in a difference in leg length and in extra rolling—one leg will tend to roll and move out (abduction) while the other will tend to roll and move in (adduction). One knee will hyperextend and the other will bend. These compensations are caused by the rotational component of the pelvis and are often reproduced in standing.

Placement

Sit against the wall and place a bolster lengthwise to support your spine and back. The support of the bolster will create a lift for both sides of the trunk as well as a release in the organic body that will cause the organs to feel supported from the back.

What to do

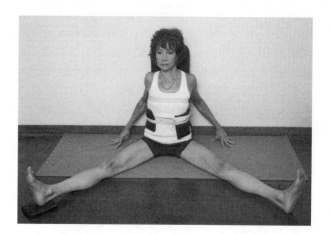

Extend the legs from the inner groin to the heels and press the back of the legs down. Press the finger tips down to lift the sides of the trunk and adjust your ribs. The convex ribs compact in and the concave ribs lift and spread as both legs extend.

Note

Adapt your hand position to lift the trunk and to open the armpit and chest. You can decentralize the hands to bring evenness and freedom to the asymmetries.

Variation 2: Facing a Chair

Props

Mat, chair, blankets.

Benefits

The pressure of the palm of the hands on the chair seat brings stability, helps extend the front, back, and sides of the spine, and induces the correction of the asymmetric ribs.

Placement

Sit facing a chair in dandasana. Spread one leg at a time to the side. Align both the inner and the outer edges of the legs. Place and spread the palms of both hands in line with the shoulders on the chair seat, and extend your arms. Look straight ahead with both eyes.

What to Do

Extend the inside of the legs from the inner groin to the inner heels, and draw the little toe and the outer heel toward the outer hip. Compact and firm both hips, root and spread the sitting bones, and lengthen the sacrum and the tailbone as the pubic bone lifts up and the abdomen moves back toward the spine. Push down both hands equally, extend the arms, and lift both sides of the trunk. From the extension of the arms, move the outer shoulder blades in and roll the shoulders down. From the pressure of the right hand, compact the convex ribs in and lift the front side of the chest. From the pressure of your left hand, extend the arm and lift the ribs up and away from the hip, focusing on the floating ribs of the concave side. To fill the flat side, move the front ribs to the back and spread the back ribs away from the spine. Push down again with both hands to lengthen the front, the back, and the sides of the trunk. Release the legs one at a time and bring them together in dandasana.

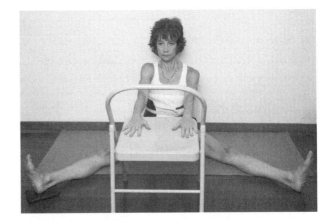

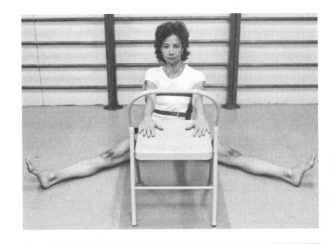

Variation 3: Facing the Wall

Props

Mat, wall, rope.

Benefit

This variation works with the extension of the inner legs, which is fundamental for the stretching of the spine.

Placement

Place a mat on the floor with the wide side along the wall. Sit in dandasana facing the wall. Extend the right leg out, and then the left leg, making sure they are at the same angle. Touch the wall with the inner edges of your ankles and feet—the wall provides proprioception and feedback at the inner heels that causes them to lengthen and ground and thereby activate the inner leg and groin, as well as the core. If you have wall ropes, hold the middle or higher ropes with each hand. Otherwise, lift both arms up, as in urdhva hastasana, and press your palms against the wall. Gradually bring the hands down to the floor in line with the shoulders. You may also hold the edge of a counter or an exercise bar to extend and pull the arms.

What to Do

Extend both legs, stretch the soles of your feet, lower your thighs, and firm the outer hips. Distribute the weight and root both sitting bones. Move the inner edges of the feet to the wall, press and ground the inner ankles, extend the toes and legs from the inner groin to the inner ankles, lengthen the sacrum and tailbone down, and then lift the pubic bone. Pull the ropes simultaneously to lift the sides of the body. From this position, adjust the ribs as needed. If the convex side is on the right, pull the rope with the right hand and bring the ribs and outer shoulder blade in while the front of the chest lifts.

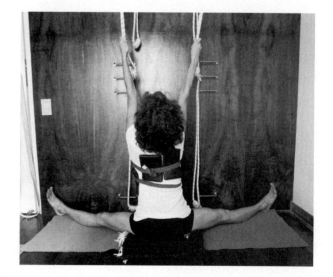

If the concave side is on the left, hold the left rope higher than the right. Pull the rope, lift the left ribs away from the hip, and spread the side ribs away from the spine. Stay in this position while pulling the ropes with equal force. If you become tired, rest the hands with rounded fingers next to the hips.

If your lumbar spine is curved, work from the legs. Press the inner edge of the feet, extend the legs, and rotate the segment of the spine where the vertebrae deviate in.

Note

Both sitting bones are spread and grounded to the sides in line with the heels. Observe and adjust if one leg rolls out. Use the proper height to sit; your weight should be centered over the sitting bones.

SWASTIKASANA: AUSPICIOUS ASANA

Props

Mat, blankets, chair, wall, pads, wooden wedge.

Benefits

This is a cross-legged position that compacts and stabilizes the hip joint. The position provides a solid base of support for the buttocks and pelvic floor. The wall supports both sides of the back and helps you maintain the posture longer with relative ease.

Placement

Sit on two blankets in dandasana. Bend your right leg, and place the foot under your left thigh. Do the same on the opposite side. The shinbone crosses in the center, and the outer edges of your feet touch the ground. Put your hands next to your hips, thumbs facing back and fingers forward. Touch the floor evenly with your fingertips. At the end, rest your palms up on your thighs.

Note

If one sitting bone is receiving more weight, place a pad under the opposite side. Experiment with different hand positions to create stability for the shoulders. The fingers can face forward and the thumbs back, or the thumbs face forward and the fingers backward.

What to Do

Spread and adjust your sitting bones with your hands. If one sitting bone is closer to the midline, adjust twice on that side to ensure that the bone and the flesh spread and create a space for the tailbone. Adjust the legs so the crossed shinbones are in line with the navel and the root of the legs moves toward the socket. Compact both outer hips in by firming the sides of the legs as the thighs lower. Push down equally with all of your fingers, and balance your weight between the front and the back of your body. While the sitting bones spread and press the floor, the outer hips move in, the thighs release down, and the sides of the spine and trunk rise.

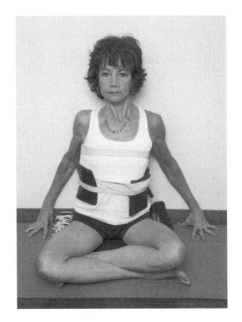

Uncross your legs and recross them while switching top and bottom positions. Observe what happens to the pelvis. If the legs are moving above the pelvis, add an extra blanket to increase the height and base of support. If you are unable to get into this position, do baddha konasana (bound angle) instead.

Variation 1: With a Chair

Props

Mat, wall, blankets, chair.

Placement

Place both hands on the chair seat, as in the upavistha konasana variation. Use the hands as levers to lift the spine and adjust the sides of the spine. Root the top of the thighs to the socket as both sides of the trunk elongate. From the pressure of each hand, move the convex ribs in and lengthen the concave. Lift the front, back, and sides of the trunk and spine.

What to Do

Cross the middle of the shin bones. From the pressure of the hands extend the legs and lift the trunk. Press the convex hand and move the ribs in. Press the concave hand and broaden the ribs. Press both hands and broaden the chest.

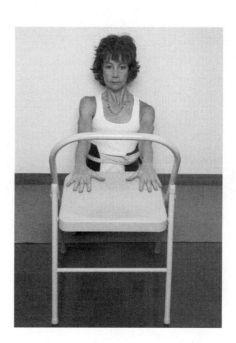

Variation 2: With Back to a Chair

Place a mat on the floor by the wall and the chair back to the wall. Sit on two or more folded blankets with your back against the chair seat, and fold the legs in swastikasana.

Cup your fingers and rest them on your thighs. Lift the sides of your trunk and your chest.

Benefits

The sharp angle of the chair provides a firm support for the thoracic vertebrae and the middle of the chest.

What to Do

Press the outer edges of the feet and bring the outer hips in. Press the fingers evenly on the floor, just behind the thighs, and lift and slightly coil the middle and upper back on the chair as both sides of the waist move back.

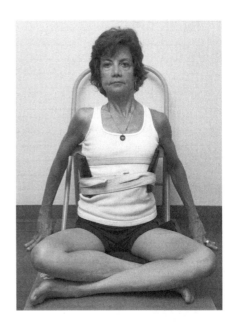

Variation 3: With Back Support

Props

Mat, blankets, wooden wedge, wooden plank, pole.

Benefits

The wooden plank, the wedge, or the pole controls the action, so that the shoulders and chest open and the spine feels stabilized and lifted.

Placement

Sit on two or more blankets in swastikasana. Hold a pole or wooden plank under the upper arms behind your back—if you are using the wooden plank, turn it so that the flat side is against the back.

What To Do

Repeat the actions from the previous variation. Move the outer elbows in and roll the upper arms from the inside out as the back of the upper arms lengthen down. Coil from the convex side and open the front of the chest. The concave side lifts and broadens as the outer elbow moves in.

Ground both sitting bones, lower your thighs, lift your ribs away from your hips, and roll your shoulders back and down while the chest lifts and spreads. Change to a cross-legged position.

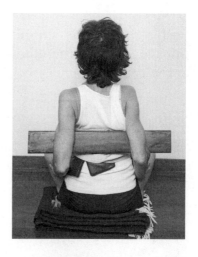

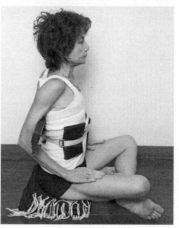

Variation 4: Seated with a Pole

Props

Mat, two or three blankets, wall, a long pole, pads.

Benefits

Stabilization of the shoulder blades.

Placement

Fold three blankets and place the pole next to them. Sit on the center of the blankets in dandasana. Move into swastikasana. If your curve is on the right thoracic spine or is a double curve, hold the pole from the back with the left hand high and the right hand low. Return to dandasana. Switch sides but continue holding the pole with the same hand position.

Note

For the best action of the shoulder blade on the concave side, lift the elbow in and up toward the ceiling.

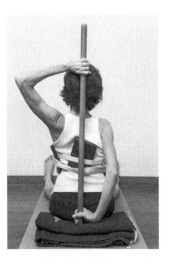

What to Do

Hold the pole, roll the shoulders back and down, and lift both sides of the trunk. The outer shoulder blade on the convex side moves down as your right elbow moves down, the left side will rise as your left elbow moves up. The elbows move in opposition. The middle of the chest bone lifts and spreads. Release your arms and feel your breath on both sides of your chest for a couple of minutes.

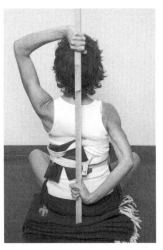

Variation 5: Holding the Pole with Both Hands

Placement

Spread the legs and press the feet on the back legs of the chair. Hold the pole with both hands parallel to the floor. Gradually lift the pole up with the arms next to the ears. Spread the hands to the side to bring more freedom for the chest and ribs.

What To Do

Extend the legs and press the back of the thighs and heels down as the sides of the trunk lift.

Note

In case the arms get tired, release the hands back to the chair.

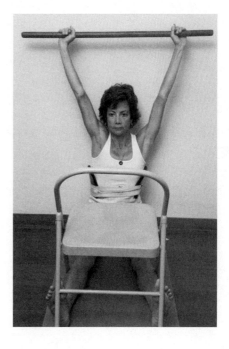

VIRASANA: HERO

Props

Mat, bolster or blankets, chair.

Benefits

The position of the legs in virasana stabilizes the sacrum and the hip joint, grounds the pelvis, and lifts the lumbar spine. For lumbar scoliosis it is very helpful, as the vertebrae begin to extend and create the proper lumbar curve, bringing the weight to the knobs of the sitting bones and roots so that the lumbar spine elongates. This posture is therapeutic for the knees, ankles, and feet (under the guidance of a teacher), and it can be done after eating.

Placement

Fold a blanket in half and place it on the mat below the chair. Kneel on the blanket with your knees together and your inner ankles slightly farther apart than your hips. Point your toes back, and touch the floor with the tops of your feet. Grasp your calf muscles and rotate them outward. Sit on a bolster, horizontal block, or blankets. Use the chair to support the back. If your knees hurt or your lower back becomes rounded, sit on the bolster with your legs together. Place both hands on the soles of your feet and then on your knees.

Note

The desired height of the prop will depend on how far the pelvis is off the ground.

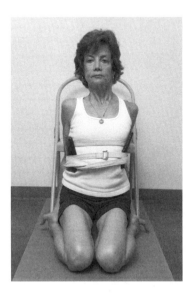

What to Do

Roll the inner thighs in, lift the pubic bone up and lengthen the tailbone as both sides of the lumbar spine lift. Roll the shoulders away from the ears and spread both sides of the chest. Use the hands to guide the ribs.

Spread the sitting bones, press them down, move the top of the sacrum in and the lower back (lumbar) up, move the root of the legs in, firm the outer legs and soften the groin, and roll the inner thigh in. Cup the hands on the soles of the feet and roll the shoulders down. Roll the outer shoulder blades in and the convex side in. Place both hands on the knees and coil the chest. Extend the arms and lift up. Lengthen the inner edges of the arms and lift the ribs. Compact the convex side in and lengthen the concave side. Relax the diaphragm and breathe on both sides. Lower the arms and release the legs in dandasana.

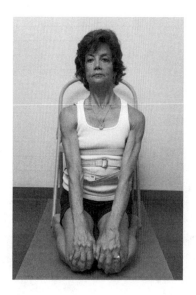

Variation 1: Holding a Pole

Props

Mat, bolster, pole, blankets.

Benefit

The pole provides traction for the spine and elongates the back, front, and sides of the trunk. It also organizes the postural muscles to firm the shoulder blades and lift the spine.

Placement

Sit in virasana or vajrasana (heels together), and hold the pole from the back of the arms. The arms wrap around the pole.

What to Do

Hold the pole and pull it tight as the shoulders move away from the ears. Bring the protracted shoulder blade (convex side) in and the retracted shoulder blade (concave) out. With the pole across the back, press the front side of the arm of the convex side to move the ribs in. Move the concave ribs toward the pole. Bring the waist and the lumbar spine back to avoid the banana shape. Lift the trunk up by moving the sitting bones down. Bring the convex side in and spread the concave. Align the back of the head with the tailbone. The middle of the chest spreads to the right and to the left, and the clavicles are broadened.

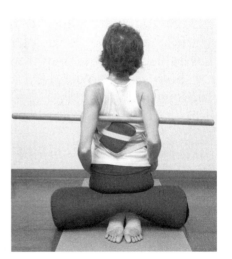

7

Forward, Lateral, Abdominal, and Back Extensions

This chapter offers a modified selection of this very important asana group. To view the traditional asanas and their proper sequence and variations, please refer to *Light on Yoga* by B. K. S. Iyengar.

FORWARD EXTENSIONS

The forward extension postures are a group of asanas that bring elongation to the spine while the torso folds forward. Keeping the solid foundation of sitting that you learned from dandasana, and the proprioception (feeling) from one's contact to the floor mentioned in the previous chapter, the body is now prepared to move in the forward dimension. The spine deals with the compressive forces caused by the body's folding, and the tensile forces caused by the forward elongation of the torso. For the health of the vertebrae and to elongate both sides of the torso, the yoga protocol focuses on the tensile forces. This group of postures keeps the body simultaneously active and resting: There is a continuous forward direction against the pull of gravity while the abdominal organs soften and lengthen to support the spine.

In the asymmetric spine, the forward extension postures teach both sides of the body to extend and to unwind the torques, compressions, and droppings. With the help of gravity, the protruded rib cage (posterior convexity) is able to move in toward the spine and move down toward the floor as the front of the spine extends forward. Opposite, on the flat side (posterior concavity), the action is to lengthen and spread the ribs. Breathing plays an important role: Exhalation serves as a tool to bring the convex side down, and inhalation brings fullness to the concave ribs. On both sides of the abdomen, organs are soft but not loose, moving back toward the spine to support the back concavities and to engage the core muscles.

Props

Mats, wall, ropes, blankets, bolster, pillows, pads, belts, chair, wooden wedges, pole or a broom, and a table. The preparation of props requires time and thought. My suggestion is to organize all the main props near you.

Benefits

Study these forward-seated postures and you will learn how to bring sensitivity to yourself. Observe the pushes, pulls, and collapses that occur between both sides, and the difference of weight and contact to the floor between sitting bones. One side will feel light and the other will feel heavy, and one side will move closer to the centerline. Observe how the feet and legs extend symmetrically. Which leg tends to roll out or in? Which knee flexes or hyperextends? How do the positions of the head and chin bone affect the neck and thoracic spine?

What to Do

Lift the pelvis with folded blankets or a bolster to provide the proper extension of the lumbar spine and to improve the posture. If the knee is coming off the floor, add extra blankets. Spread the legs and arms mat-width apart (decentralized) to create length, balance, and stability and to release compressions. Use chairs or blocks to elevate the hands and upper arms and to create space and elongation on both sides of the rib cage, chest, and spine. The principle in the forward extension is to fold forward from the hip joints, rooting the head of the femur into the hip socket, firming the outer hip, and separating the torso and spine from the legs. The scoliotic spine has to learn how to elongate from the back, front, and sides, and mainly on the compressive pulls of the curves. Work contralaterally—this means relating both sides in a crossed pattern. For instance, in janushirasana (head to knee) full forward extension, move one side (ribs) to the opposite leg; this also includes the turning of the head. The twisted position unwinds torques and asymmetries of the ribs, especially on the convex side.

Caution

It is important to support the concave side and areas with blankets, pillows, or pads. The underneath support of the props will prevent these areas from collapsing further. Additionally, do not dome the ribs, compress the vertebral bodies of the spine, or cave the chest. In case of skeletal pathologies (knees, vertebrae, or decreased bone density), consult your physician prior to attempting these asanas.

PASCHIMOTTANASANA: FORWARD EXTENSION OF THE BACK

Variation 1A: With a Chair

Props

Mat, blankets, pillows, chair, wall.

Benefits

This symmetrical forward-extension posture offers a midline orientation and reference to the core: it tones the abdominal organs, elongates and tones the extensors (back muscles) and flexors (abdominal muscles), soothes the nervous system as the brain rests toward the support of gravity or a prop, and softens the digestive organs. The hands on the chair create the proper action for both sides of the trunk and chest to lift and to correct from the compressive pulls created from the asymmetries.

Placement

Sit in dandasana facing a chair. Place your hands on the chair seat and in line with the shoulders. Press down with the hands to lift the chest. Keeping the spine lifted, tilt the pelvis forward and hold onto the sides of the chair with straight arms. Pull the chair and lift the middle of the chest, keeping the back long. Draw the spine in as you lift the front of your body. Add an extra lift on the convex side.

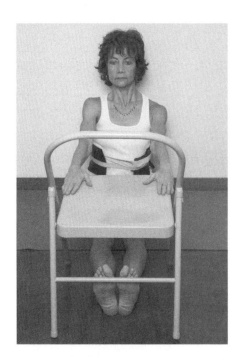

Hold the back of the chair, bring both sides of the rib cage forward, lengthen the front of the spine, and rest the forehead on the chair—place a folded blanket or a bolster on the chair seat if necessary. Maintain the arms extended in line with the ears to lengthen and spread the upper ribs. To come out, make both legs stiff and extend the sides of the trunk, lifting up to a seated position in dandasana. Look to the front with a soft gaze as you observe both sides and the breath.

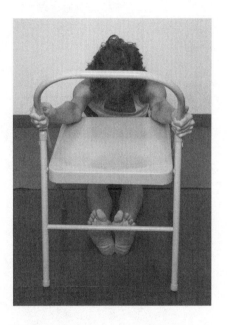 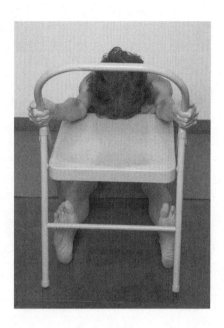

Variation 1B: Chair Adho Mukha Paschimottanasana

Props

Mat, chair, blankets.

Placement

Sit on the edge of the chair, extend the legs as in dandasana. Place a folded blanket on your lap to help fill the concave side as you extend the trunk forward over the legs. Hold the feet, and gradually release the palms of the hands to the floor.

What to Do

Extend the legs and press the heels down. Lengthen the inner groin to the inner heels. The outer heels pull back toward the outer hips as the trunk extends forward from the sides of the ribs. The crown of the head releases from the spine. The convex ribs move in and the concave ribs lengthen and fill from the front. The middle chest descends toward the legs.

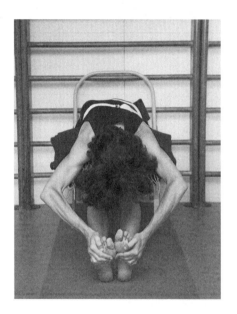

Note

Decentralize the position; spread the legs apart.

Variation 2: With a Plank or Pole

Props

Mat, blankets, pillows, a wooden plank, pole, or broom.

Benefits

This asana offers a midline orientation and reference to center; the plank adds the elongation of both sides of the rib cage, brings extension to the front of the spine, tones the abdominal organs and back muscles, and soothes the nervous system as the brain and digestive organs rest toward gravity.

Placement

Place the wooden plank at the front edge of the mat. Sit on two or more blankets in dandasana. Check on the foundation: Determine if one sitting bone receives more weight and/or if it is closer to the medial line. Adjust, spread, and distribute the weight between both sitting bones. Fold one blanket lengthwise and place it on the convex side leg, and increase the height on the concave side. Extend both legs evenly, lift both arms up in urdhva hasta dandasana, and bring the trunk forward. Hold the outer edges of the plank, extend the arms, and lift both sides of the rib cage as the chest and the spine go up. This is the first phase of the extension. Learn how to bring elongation to the spine from this stage. Gradually continue with the extension of both sides of the rib cage, tilting from the pelvis, and bring the torso forward. Bend and lift the elbows, and pull the plank as the trunk further extends.

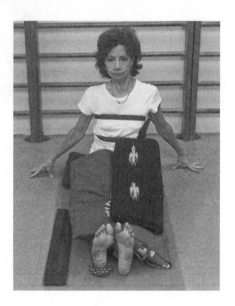

What to Do

As you extend the legs, press the heels down and lengthen the feet. Lift both arms and lengthen the sides, come forward and take hold of the plank that is bracing the heels. Pull the prop, firm the legs, lift the pubic bone, bring both sides of the abdomen in toward the spine, and extend the sides of the trunk forward as the spine moves in. As you extend forward, release the front of the body on the support. Move the thick ribs (convex) in and touch the support with the chest. As the concave side ribs lengthen, move back and spread. Both sides of the abdomen move toward the spine.

To come out, release the hands, extend the spine and legs, reach toward the top of the head, and return to dandasana.

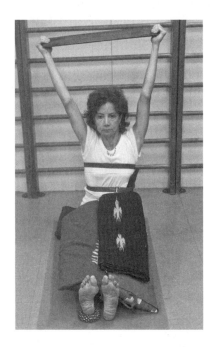

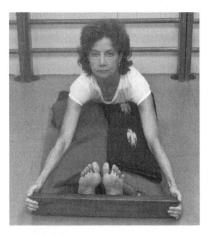

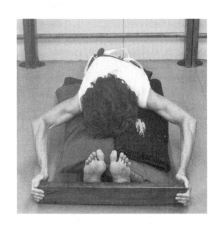

Variation 3: Legs and Arms Apart

Decentralized

Props

Mat, blankets, wooden plank or pole, blocks.

Benefits

The decentralized position of the limbs is very helpful for the stability of both sides, and it facilitates the correction and release of the asymmetric rib cage. It is an important modification that relieves back pain and tightness. Overall, the asana provides space and mobility for the asymmetric spine to extend and to open the closed spaces in the front.

Placement

Sit on two or more blankets in dandasana. Have a pole near you; it can be in front of the feet or on the floor next to the hip. Move the legs apart in line with the outer edges of the mat. The feet should be parallel and the toes pointing upward. The middle of the thighs are centered on the knees, shinbone, and center of the feet. Press the hands on the floor or on blocks to lift the torso. Take hold of the pole and bring it to the soles of the feet in front of the heel. Hold the pole evenly with both hands. Extend the legs and pull with the hands. This is the first phase of the extension. The thoracic spine will move in and forward to a full forward extension as the front of the body elongates.

Lift the pubic bone, bring the abdomen in, and extend forward from the sides of the ribs. Come out of the pose by firming the legs, engaging the abdomen, extending the trunk, releasing the plank, and sitting in dandasana.

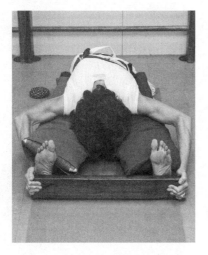
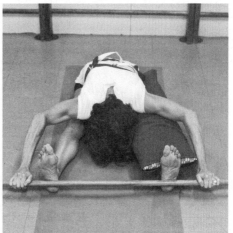

Variation 4: With Blocks

If Variation 3 is not possible, try replacing the plank with two tall blocks.

Props

Mat, blankets, three blocks.

Benefits

This is an alternative to the plank. The height and position of the blocks will vary accordingly.

Placement

Sit on the blankets in dandasana; place the blocks next to each foot or leg and position a third one for the head. The blocks are to be placed at the same height.

What to Do

From dandasana, lift the arms in urdhva has-tasana from the sides of the rib cage. Move the shoulder blades in and down, elongate the trunk forward from the hip joint, and place both hands on the blocks. Press the hands and lengthen the sides, moving the lower ribs away from the hips. As you come forward, widen the blocks and bring the thick side in as you bring the side that drops (concave) back and out. Move the thoracic spine in and spread the chest. Extend the trunk forward and rest the forehead on the third block. The back of the head should be in line with the spine, and the armpits and chest should be in line with the shoulders.

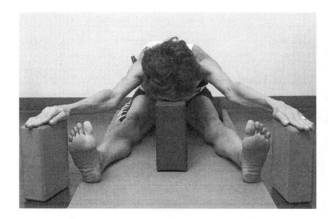

Note

To extend the thoracic spine and reduce the convexity of the rib cage, place the chin bone on the block.

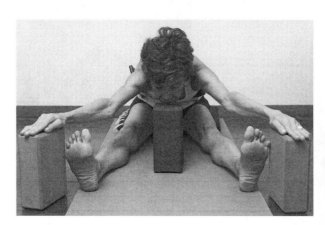

EKA PADA PASCHIMOTTANASANA

Placement

Sit on two folded blankets in dandasana with the legs mat-width apart. Place two thin pillows or fold a couple of blankets for each leg and an extra lengthwise-folded blanket for the concave side. Hold a pole or plank and bring the trunk into a forward extension over the right leg. Place the plank on the heels.

What to Do

Move and lengthen the right rib cage and the chest toward the pillow. If this is your convex side, this movement will undo the back convexity and dome shape. Move the right elbow up and the shoulder blade in.

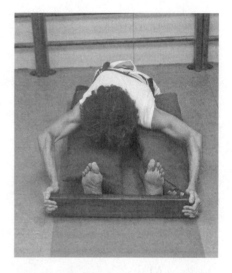

Note

The support for the crown of the heels and sitting bone prevented that side from rolling and dropping toward the floor.

On the left side (concave), the support is higher, and the goal is to bring the right ear to the left leg. This creates thoracic vertebrae derotation and elongation. The armpit continues to move forward from the middle of the chest, giving a feeling of a symmetrical back.

The overall effects of decentralizing the limbs, with the addition of the wooden plank, allow the motion of the thoracic vertebrae to lengthen and the ribs to self-correct. I have been integrating this in my personal practice.

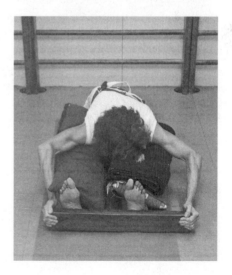

CHAIR JANU SIRSASANA: HEAD-TO-KNEE

Variation 1: Concave Phase

Benefits

The extension phase of this forward-bending posture is very important for the spinal traction because it tones the back muscles and the abdominal organs, and addresses the length of both sides of the rib cage. The hands on the chair serve as vectors from which the weight between both sides is adjusted.

Props

Mat, blankets, chair.

Note

If the bent knee is lifted, add an extra blanket to sit on.

Placement

Have a chair facing you on the front side of the mat. Sit on the two blankets, and extend both legs in dandasana. Open the buttocks—with the hands spreading the muscles and skin. Adjust the chair so it is near the level of the middle shinbones. Bend the right leg, bring the right foot into janu sirsasana, and roll the outer thigh down.

Lift both arms up as in urdhva hastasana (urdhva hasta janu sirsasana) with the palms facing each other. Maintain the lift of both sides of the rib cage, and place the palms of the hands on the chair seat in line with the shoulders. Adjust the chair, if necessary, to extend the arms and for the pressure of the hands to lift the side body. Hold the side of the chair and pull the arms, and look up by moving the spine in and spreading both sides of the chest. The chair serves as a platform from which the chest lifts. To come out, release the arms and legs to dandasana.

What to Do

From dandasana, bend the right leg, and press the sole of the foot on the upper thigh. Lift the pubic bone and the abdomen back toward the spine, lengthen the sacrum, and move the upper part in while keeping the tailbone down as the lumbar spine lifts. Lift both arms and lengthen both sides of the rib cage. Continue with the extension of the trunk; press the hands to lift both sides of the rib cage, bringing the outer shoulder blade in and the shoulders away from the ears. Spread and lift both sides of the chest. Add extra pressure on one hand to bring the convex ribs in, and then do the same with the opposite hand, lifting and spreading the ribs. Lift both sides and the chest.

Note

For a full forward extension, slide the chair out and place a blanket or bolster horizontally on the chair seat. While holding the back of the chair, rest the forehead on the blanket.

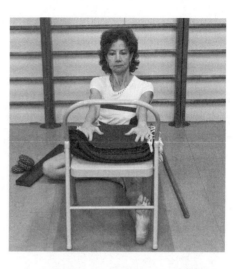

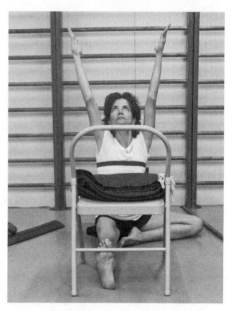

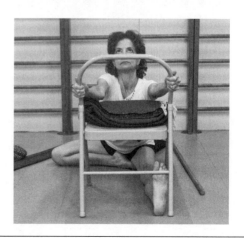

MODIFIED JANU SIRSASANA

Variation 2: With a Plank

Note

The use of the wooden plank requires skill and extra help from an assistant or teacher. If the final position is not possible, replace the plank with two blocks that are placed on either side of the extended leg, belts, or a chair.

Props

Mat, blankets, a wooden plank, pole, or broom, belt, pad, wall, chair, bolster.

Benefits

This is a very important posture for scoliosis because it includes extension, flexion, lateral flexion, and rotation. It tones the legs, the back muscles, the flexors, and the core muscles, the abdominal organs, and the kidneys. The rotation component of the posture works on the organic body and the asymmetries of the ribs, and it releases holdings in the postural muscles. The pad placed on the back brings proprioception and feedback to the back ribs.

Note

To address the forward extension on the concave side, it is important to fold an extra blanket between the thigh and pelvis. The blankets are used as a support to lift the drops and collapses.

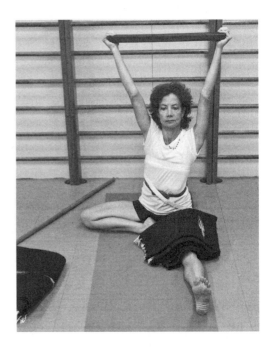

Note

The placement of the plank from the sitting position might be a challenge for some; in this case, have the plank next to the extended leg's foot and adjust it on the heel in the full forward position. The thick edge of the plank is down. If you do not have this special prop, use a pole, stick, or even a broom to pull and open the side ribs and chest.

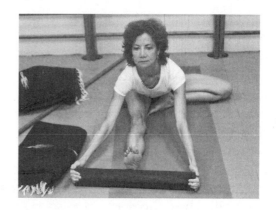

Placement

Have the props next to you. Sit on two folded blankets in dandasana, and adjust the sitting position for equal distribution of weight. Study this sitting position and observe how both sitting bones receive the weight. Sense how the pelvis makes contact with the blankets. Position the wooden plank next to you on the left side next to the left leg. Bend the right leg and place the right heel near the perineum, with the toes of the right foot in contact with the left inner thigh like in vrkshasana (tree posture). The outer heel of the straight leg is in line with the left outer hip. Fold one or more blankets on the top of the left thigh to support the concave side and the convex ventral rib. The height will vary according to the degree of the curve and your experience. To soothe this asymmetric extension, you can add a bolster on the shin bone to support the forehead.

Now, the extended leg is rooted and aligned. The outer heel is in line with the outer hip. Next, soften the abdominal organs to rotate the right side of the waist toward the left. Take the plank or pole and bring it to the left heel. This can be done by extending the arms over the head or by adding the plank after being in the posture. A chair can also replace the plank if the position is not possible.

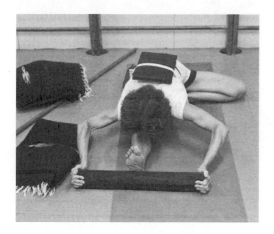

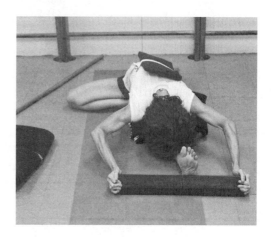

Hold the plank with both hands, lift the arms up, and look up. Maintaining the extension of both sides of the trunk, lift the chest, begin tilting the pelvis (flexion) forward, and move both sides of the rib cage (torso) forward over the left leg. As the body extends forward, place the plank or pole next to the heel of the left foot, bend and lift both elbows away from each other, lengthen both sides of the rib cage and chest, and arrive at full forward extension. The lower abdomen is soft but not dropped: it recedes back toward the spine so the lumbar spine is able to lengthen. Rest the chin bone on the support. The position of the chin helps the extension of the thoracic spine and opens it in the front while moving the convex torso down. The protruding ribs move down with each exhalation, and the concave ribs fill and lengthen with each inhalation. Maintain the extension of the leg and trunk, come to the full forward position, and turn the right ear toward the left shin bone. This will bring a counter rotation for the thoracic curve on the right side. Stay there as long as you can, being careful not to strain. Let the breathing be natural. To come out of the posture, release the right leg, and bring the legs to dandasana.

Note

With practice, the bent leg of janu sirsasana moves farther back, creating an obtuse angle with the toe touching the upper left thigh. It externally rotates, but both sides of the trunk remain facing front. In the case of the lumbar curve, the oblique angle helps the derotation of the vertebrae as the back leg gently pulls and rotates the lumbar spine. In the case of a left lumbar curve, the right leg works to derotate the curve as it gently pulls and rotates the pelvis.

What to Do

As the right foot presses the inner left thigh, compact both hips internally and rotate the right thigh. Hold the plank and lift both arms up, lengthen the sides of the ribs, lift the chest, and look up. The pubic bone lifts up, the abdomen recedes back, the sacrum shifts inward, and the lumbar spine elongates. Come forward from the tilt of the pelvis as both sides of the rib cage lengthen away from the pelvis. Grip firmly the outer edges of the plank, lift the elbows up, and stabilize the outer shoulder blades in. Lengthen the right side, bring the ribs in toward the left side, and rest both sides

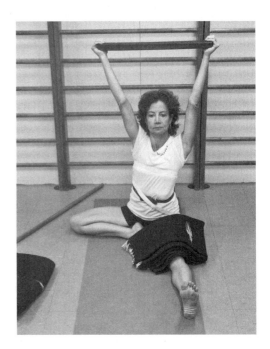

of the trunk on the left leg. During the exhalation, extend the chin bone on the shin and bring the convex ribs in and down. During inhalation, as the concave back ribs fill with air, turn the head and move the right ear toward the left shin as both sides of the trunk extend. Bring the waist back toward the spine and soften the abdominal organs as the torso extends over the left leg. To come out, firm the extended leg, pull the plank in to come to a concave phase of the posture, and lift both sides of the chest. Bring the arms up and release the hands from the prop, releasing the right leg and sitting in dandasana. Observe both sides and the breathing.

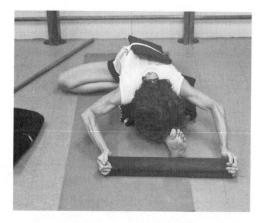

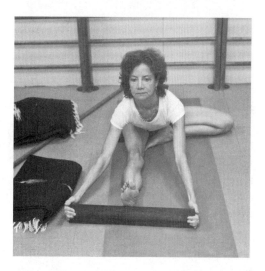

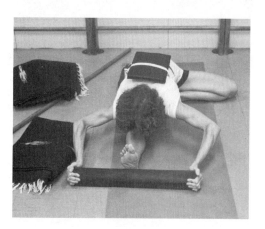

LATERAL EXTENSIONS/ROTATION

This group of asanas addresses the spinal extension and rotation—the best treatment for the three-dimensional pattern of scoliosis.

Suggestions

- For scoliosis, the twists cannot be the same on both sides; each side will require a different mechanical action. It is important to know where the convexities and concavities (right, left, back, and front) are and the nature of the curve(s). Once you become sensitive to the pattern, your inner intelligence will emerge and help you guide your exercises with the proper modifications.
- Lengthen and create a space in both sides of the rib cage first, then soften the belly to rotate.
- Adjust both sides of the rib cage by stabilizing the convex side with the action of the outer shoulder blade moving in and the ribs compacting toward the spine. Elongate the concave side by moving the outer shoulder blade in, lifting the ribs away from the pelvis, and modifying the arm position. Once you practice this action, the arms will work symmetrically.
- Initiate the rotation from the limbs (appendicular) as a lever to rotate the spine.
- Explore rotating segmentally (pelvis, chest, neck, and head) and fluidly. Use the eyes to add another dimension to the twist; look up to lift the chest. When twisting to the convex side, look up and move the head back. This will bring the ribs in.
- Work with repetition and add motion to the twists to bring mobility and fluidity to the organs, fascia, ligaments, and joints on both sides.
- Do not push or compress the spine.

Caution

- Avoid rigid patterns of holding in the twists. Additionally, holding the breath creates rigidity in the nervous system.
- Do not look down when rotating because doing so will cave the chest and depress the posture.
- Do not reinforce the asymmetry; keep your awareness sharp so that both sides are constantly aiming for length.
- Rest when the mind can no longer focus. Learn from the asanas on how to gain awareness; do not practice mechanically.

BHARADVAJASANA: BHARADVAJA, A SAGE

The following variations of this posture are to be done according to the individual's curves in order for the proper modification to be addressed. The props can be used under the armpit to inhibit the convexity of the ribs and to induce the retracted ribs to spread toward the contact. For the short concave side, you could also place a block underneath the left armpit to induce the retracted ribs to spread toward the block. For the convex side, the block should be underneath the armpit to induce the protruded ribs to move in.

Variation 1

Props

Mat, blankets, two blocks.

Benefits

This seated twist increases the mobility of the organs, extends the trunk, and promotes proper action for concave and convex sides. It addresses the thoracic and lumbar segments and the three-dimensional pattern of the curve.

Placement

Sit on two blankets in dandasana. Bend the knees and place the feet beside the left hip, with the left instep resting in the right arch. Both sitting bones should be down on the blankets. Cup both hands behind your back, and press the fingers equally to lift both sides of the rib cage. If the concave side is on the left, place a block underneath the left armpit to induce the retracted ribs to spread toward the block. Lift and twist the spine to the right, and place the left palm on the floor outside the right thigh. Hold the thigh with the left hand, and place the right hand back near the left buttock. After structuring the posture, begin the twist to the right (or convex) side.

Release the arms and legs and extend the legs into dandasana. Repeat the pose a couple of times to increase the mobility of the torso.

Note

If the left is your convex side (right thoracic curve), hold the right side firmly with the left hand to induce the ribs to come in. As you read these instructions, it is important that you remember that my left side is my concave side and my right is convex: adjust accordingly for a right thoracic curve.

If the hips are uneven, increase the height of the seat and back hand.

What to Do

Hold the outer right side tightly with the left hand, and cup the right hand behind the left buttock or on a block. During inhalation, lift both sides of the rib cage up with a strong grip; during exhalation, twist to the right, look up to lift the chest, and move the head slightly backward to bring the convex ribs in as the left ribs (concave) lengthen. Unwind the twist, release the arms and legs back to dandasana, and change sides.

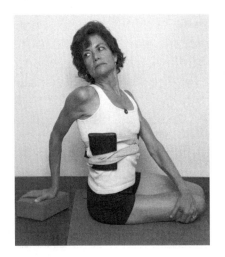

Left side

Add an extra block under the left armpit to induce the ribs to spread. Pull the left side tight with your right hand and lengthen both sides of the waist. Spread the ribs toward the block and move the convex ribs. Lift up, exhale, and twist. To release, straighten the legs in dandasana.

Variation 2: At a Wall

Props

Mat, wall, three blankets or a bolster, two blocks, pads, belts. The pad is an additional tool to bring proprioception to the back body, while the block brings sensitivity to the ribs. For the lumbar curve, allow the sitting bone to slide over the edge of the bolster or blanket. The hip will gravitate down and away from the ribs.

Benefits

The wall is a useful prop for rotation. It offers the possibility to adjust the ribs and both sides.

Placement

Sit in dandasana on a bolster with the right side to the wall and the legs folded to the left. The left ankle should be placed over the arch of the right foot.

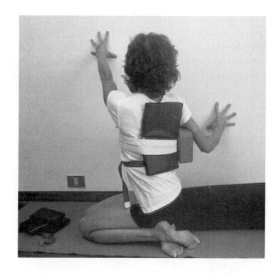

Place your fingertips on the wall and twist to the right side. Add a block under the armpit of the concave side if necessary. Extend further with the left hand up and lengthen both sides. Maintain the extension and bring the left hand on the outside of the right thigh. Have the right hand on the bolster toward the left buttock.

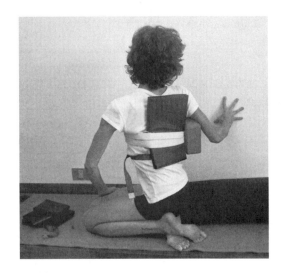

Bring the right hand behind the left buttock; use a block if this is not possible. Maintaining the imprint of the lift in the left side, bring the left hand outside the right thigh.

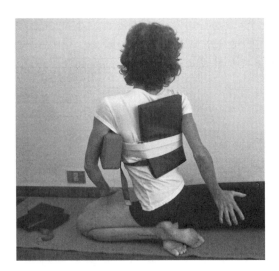

What to Do

With my left (concave) side near the wall: As the right hand spreads the back ribs and lifts both sides of the trunk, move the chest of the convex side toward the wall as both shoulder blades move in and hug the ribs. Look up to further lift the chest.

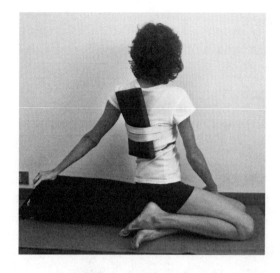

As you twist to the left, pull with the right hand and bring the left fingers back. Add the block under the armpit of the convex side ribs and squeeze it. Inhale to lift both sides and exhale as you twist the right ribs toward the left.

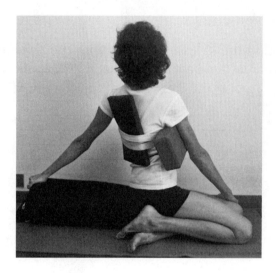

Variation 3: With a Chair

Props

Mat, chair, wall, two blocks, bolster.

Benefits

This is a very functional posture because we sit most of the time in front of computers or desks, and it is an alternative for those with more difficulties. There are various ways to sit in this asana just as there are various modalities to sit on chairs. For instance, you can straddle the chair with the legs on either side of the backrest or with the legs through the backrest, you can sit on the side of the chair with the outer hip next to the backrest, or you can sit on the diagonal corner of the chair. One hand can be on the backrest while the other hand is on the wall.

You can use a bolster between the torso and the back of the chair or wall. That will help inhibit the convexity of the ribs and invite the short side to rest on it. Each position and application will move a different segment of the spine and help organic mobility.

Placement

Sit on the side of the chair with the right (convex) side to the wall and the back of the chair. The feet are parallel and pelvis-width apart. If the feet do not touch the floor, use two blocks to support the feet. The feet and legs are the stabilizers for the rotation, so be sure that the feet, legs, and knees are even. Organize the twist from the feet.

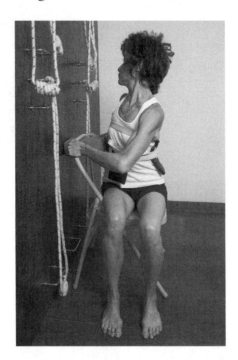

What to Do

Turn to the right and hold the back of the chair. Lift the elbows, press the feet, lift the spine up, and then twist from the belly, ribs, and chest as the eyes follow the twist. Look from the corner of the right eye.

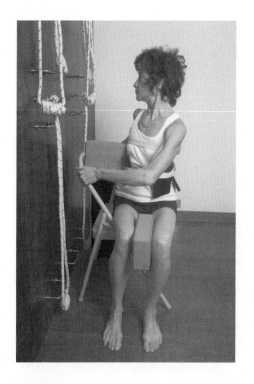

To increase the elongation of the short side, crawl with the fingers on the wall as in Variation 2. The right hand presses the chair so the convex ribs move in. Look up and move the head slightly backward. Release and come out of the posture. Change sides.

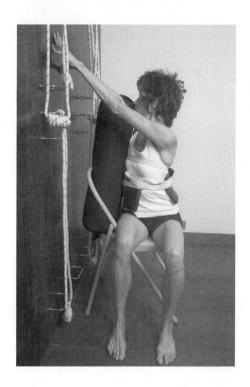

Sit on the side of the chair with your left side toward the wall. Have the legs pelvis-width apart. Press and lengthen the feet and then rotate to the left, placing both hands on the back of the chair. Move the convex ribs in with a push of the right hand.

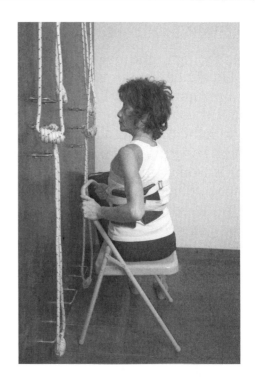

If the curve is on the left side, as the torso rotates to the left, move the abdomen to the right. Bring the lumbar spine in.

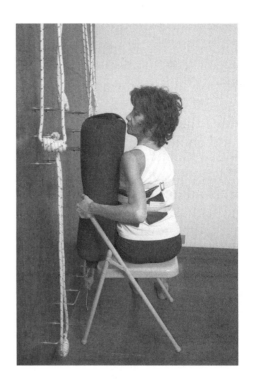

ABDOMINAL EXTENSIONS

One of the protocols in physical therapy for scoliosis is to strengthen the core. The flexors support the extensors; the front supports the back. A loose abdomen creates instability in the spine. The yoga abdominal asanas tone the abdominal muscles and organs, and lengthen the abdominal wall. For the traditional asanas, please see *Light on Yoga* by B. K. S. Iyengar.

Here I share variations of the asanas that I have found helpful for scoliosis. Remember that this work is to be done under the guidance of a teacher. Do not perform these asanas during your menstrual period or if you have any pelvic medical condition, including sacro-iliac conditions.

The extension of the legs happens from the stabilization of the hip joint. The outer hips firm in and draw back down to the floor. The head of the femur moves into the hip joint, the sacrum moves in and the pubic bone moves up, and the very bottom of the abdomen and navel lift up and move toward the spine. The inner groin moves to the inner heel, and the small toe moves to the outer heel and then to the outer hip.

Suggestions

- Before lying down, arrange all the props near you. Use blankets folded lengthwise to support both sides of the spine; do not place them up too high.
- In case of lower back pain, placing another blanket under the pelvis will help. If yours is a chronic condition, bend both legs. In the variations in the subsequent texts, a bolster will serve this purpose.
- Lie on the center of the mat; ask an assistant or teacher to help you if necessary. Support the concave areas and the lumbar spine—which tend to lift away from the floor—with blankets and pads or by elevating the feet on blocks. Support the convex areas by lifting the back ribs with pads or wedges.
- If the hip is higher on one side and lifts away from the floor, place the pad on the opposite side to balance the pelvis. The same applies with the outer shoulders.
- When using a belt, the buckle should be outside. Placing the middle of the belt on the heels addresses the skeletal line of force and back leg, whereas the belt on the ball of the feet addresses the muscles in the front of the legs. To avoid compression on the back, the crown of the heel should be in line with sitting bones.
- The extension of the legs happens from the inner groin to the inner heels and big toe. The small toe moves down, and the outer heel draws back toward the outer hip. Both hips firm in.

URDHVA PRASARITA PADASANA: UPWARD LEG EXTENSION

Variation 1

Props

Mat, wall, bolster, belt, blanket, pads, wooden wedge.

Benefits

The bolster offers proprioception for the sitting bones and the proper pelvic distribution of weight, and it allows the abdominal organs to soften and release back to the spine. The extension of the back legs increases the tone of the abdominal organs and muscles and stabilizes the hip joint.

Placement

Fold a blanket lengthwise to support both sides of the spine, including the neck and back of the head. Place the extra accessories near the mat (pads, wooden plank, bolster, and blanket). Place the wooden plank on the middle of the mat so it will be easy to grasp and adjust. The thin edge of the plank should be up. Lie down so the spine is supported by the long blanket, and adjust the plank so it is under the middle of the shoulder blades and chest; it must be in the center of the back. Look at its ends to verify its position. Bend the legs, and bring the feet off the floor and toward the abdomen. Place the bolster under the buttock bones, including the coccyx, so the pelvis is slightly suspended. Extend both arms by your sides, with the palms facing down. If one shoulder is lifting, add a pad under the opposite shoulder. Spread the hands away from the midline (decentralize) to open the upper chest and bring the shoulder blades in. Lift both legs up in a 90-degree angle (perpendicular) and move the femurs into the hip joint. Look straight to the ceiling.

If you are unable to extend the legs, place a strap on the center of the heels. Make sure the strap is even on both sides, and hold it with the elbows down and the chest open.

What to Do

Extend both legs as the outer edges of the hips move down. Lift the convex ribs up with a pad or wooden plank, and move the concave ribs down. As the belly moves toward the back, both sides of the torso elongate.

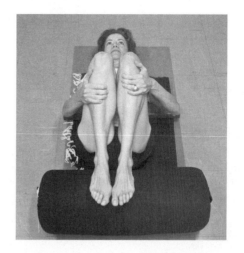

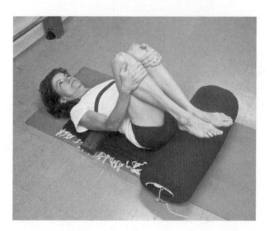

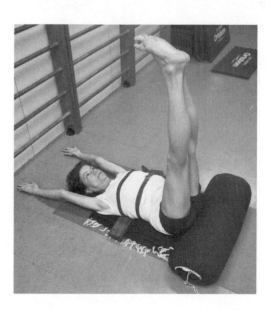

Variation 2: Legs to the Wall

Props

Wall, mat, blanket.

Benefits

This is a restorative variation of the posture, but it has profound effects on both sides of the abdomen. The abdominal muscles and organs descend and move back to support the spine.

Placement

Have a mat perpendicular to the wall. Fold a blanket lengthwise to support both sides of the spine, including the neck and back of the head. Place the extra accessories near the mat (pads, wooden plank, or wedges). Sit with the right side beside the wall, and then roll down and place both legs on the wall. You might have to attempt the position several times to get it correct. Both of the sitting bones touch the wall and the legs are perpendicular to the floor. The arms are extended over the head.

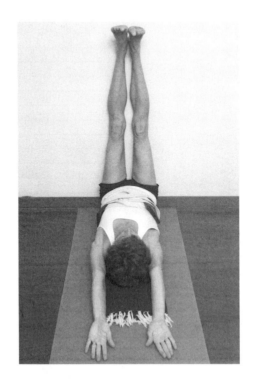

What to Do

Extend both legs on the wall, move the sitting bones to the wall, and bring the outer hips down to the floor. The navel descends toward the floor as both sides of the trunk lengthen from the extension of the arms. Roll the shoulders down and away from the ears.

Note

Decentralize the legs in case of back pain or to feel more space in the abdominal cavity.

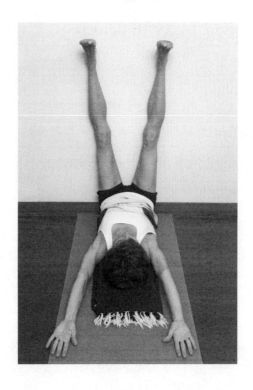

PARIPURNA NAVASANA: FULL BOAT POSE

Variation 1A: With Bent Legs

Props

Mat, blanket.

Benefits

Tone the lower abdomen and strengthen the back and kidneys.

What To Do

Sit on a folded blanket in dandasana with the hands next to the outer hips. Bend both legs and hold the back thighs with your hands. Recline back, stretch the arms, and lift the feet up perpendicular to the floor with the feet and legs together. Compact the hips, lift the ribs up, and extend the arms parallel to the floor with the palms facing each other. The arms are in line with the shoulders. If the chest is closing on one side, decentralize the arms, moving them to the side, or hold the back of the legs. Lift the legs higher. Recline the head slightly backward and look up to increase the extension as the belly moves in and up. The main thing is to balance the buttocks and lift the spine, move the convex rib in, and lift the concave rib and the chest up.

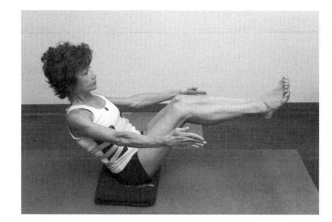

Variation 1B

If doing the exercise with the legs together is not possible, spread the feet hip-width apart.

In the full posture, the legs are extended and higher than the head. You can build the pose in stages up to the full extension of the legs with the aid of the props. Use a wall with a bolster to lean against, or sit on a folded blanket.

Variation 2: Final

Props

Mat, 16-inch belt.

Benefits

Tones the abdomen and strengthens the back muscles.

Placement

Sit on a folded blanket in dandasana and loop the belt around the balls of your feet and the lower portion of the shoulder blades. Lean against the belt, and lift the legs to a 60-degree angle. Raise the arms in line with the shoulders with the palms facing each other.

What to Do

As both sides of the back lean toward the strap, extend the legs, compact both hips, and lift the pubic bone and navel up. Raise the legs and arms together, move the upper arms back, and lift the chest. Decentralize the legs and arms. This will release pain contraction and offer space for both sides to adjust.

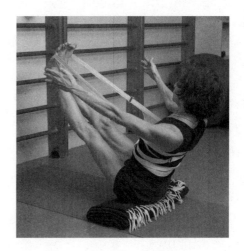

SUPTA PADANGUSTHASANA: RECLINING HAND TO BIG TOE POSTURE

Variation 1: Looped Belt and Belt on the Ball of the Feet.

Props

Wall, mat, blanket, block, 10-foot belt, short belt.

Benefits

This is an excellent asana for scoliosis because it lengthens and tones the core muscles, hip flexors, and the abdominal and hamstring muscles. The traction provided by the belt creates the proper condition for the short side to lengthen.

Placement

Place the mat on the wall. Fold a blanket lengthwise to support both sides of the back, and sit on it in the middle of the mat. Make a large loop with the 10-foot strap. Loop one end around the right outer hip, and the other end around the balls of both feet. Keep the loose end on the outside of the hip facing down toward the feet to avoid hurting the skin. Bend the right knee to the chest; the strap will wrap around the upper thigh. Make a loop in the shorter strap to place it around the ball of the right foot (increases muscular tone), and press the left foot against the wall, firm the left leg, and straighten both legs. The right leg is perpendicular to the floor. The outer edges of both hips are down. As if you are riding a horse, lower the elbows down as the shoulder blades move in, and gradually extend the arms.

What to Do

Extend the left leg, press the thighbone down, and firm the outer hips in. Keep the hips even and extend the right leg in a perpendicular line with the floor, pressing the ball of the right foot on the strap and moving the outer hips down. Lift the pubic bone up, both sides of the waist back, and the buttocks away from the lumbar spine.

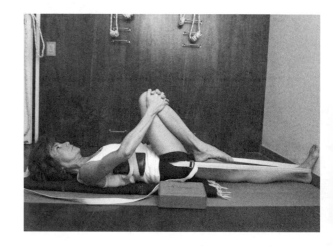

As the arms extend, roll the shoulders back and down. Draw the right outer heel toward the right hip and in line with the right sitting bone. If this is the convex side, lift the back ribs toward the ceiling, and extend the right leg while the shoulder is firmly on the floor with the outer shoulder blade in. Come out by bending the right leg, removing the belt, and being in supta tadasana to rest. Observe both sides.

For the anterior rotation of the hip caused by the lumbar curve, use a wedge or a pad to elevate the opposite hip (concave) and even both sides of the pelvis.

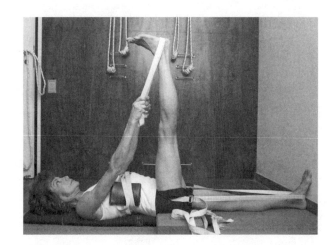

Note

An easy stage for this posture is to bend one leg with the knee over the heel. The strap on the extended leg can be used in the ball of the feet, and back on the heel or in front of the heel (arch). Feel the differences in your hip and leg.

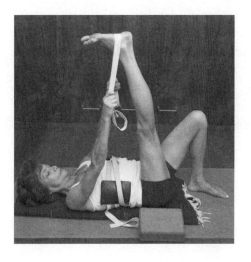

Variation 2: Leg to the Side

Repeat the first phase of the posture. Extend both legs in supta tadasana with the feet on the wall. Extend the right leg and place the strap on the ball of the foot. Fix the left leg to the wall while the right leg moves to the right side; the outer edge of the foot is parallel to the floor, working on the hip joint. The outer hip is supported by the bolster or blocks to avoid pelvic rolling. The hip is square. Feel under the left ribs to see if there is a space between the left ribs and the floor. The blanket underneath should take care of this, but if there is still a distortion in the shape, reorganize the setup; place a couple of pads or a blanket to support both sides of the spine.

Benefits

Strengthens the core and hamstrings.

What to Do

As the leg moves to the side, the outer hips compact and contact the block, and the right leg and arm extend. The shoulder rolls down and the outer shoulder blade moves in. The pubic bone lifts, and the waist spreads and moves back. The arm can be away from the midline so the upper chest can open and the shoulder blade can move in.

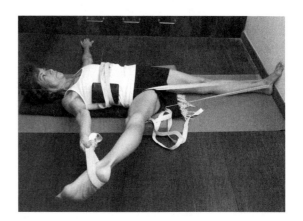

Variation 3: With Bent Leg

Placement

Bend the left leg and place the foot near the buttock bone. Bring the right leg in and place the strap on the ball of the foot. Extend the right leg at a perpendicular angle, and then move the leg to the side. This will create more space and stabilization of the hip joint.

On the concave side, when the leg moves to the side, the tendency will be for the convex hip to roll because of the weakness of the core muscles. To prevent the pelvis from rotating anteriorly, one strategy is to rotate the extended leg and move it slightly out.

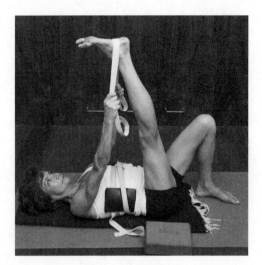
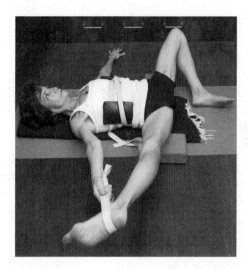

INTERMEDIATE STUDENTS

JATHARA PARIVARTANASANA: REVOLVED ABDOMINAL ASANA

Variation 1: With Legs Folded

Props

Mat, blanket, two bolsters.

Benefits

If you are unable to extend your legs, in this variation the legs are bent and supported by the bolsters. It offers the seeds of the full posture.

Placement

Lie down, with the spine and lumbar region supported with a blanket. Place two vertical bolsters next to the outer hips. Bend the legs; take the feet off the floor and close to the abdomen. Extend the arms in a T-shape, and roll the shoulders down. Exhale and bring the legs to the left hand as they rest on the bolster. Come up. Exhale and move the legs to the right hand. Come up to the center, extend the legs, and rest.

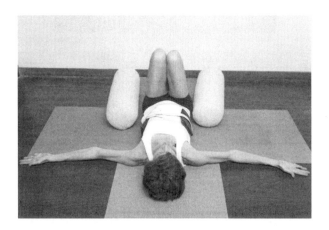 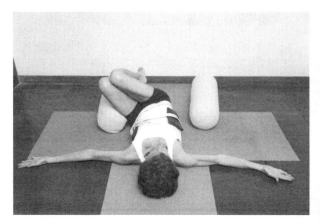

Variation 2

Props

Mat, blanket, one bolster.

Benefits

The elevation of the pelvis on the bolster helps to soften the abdominal organs and diaphragm, resulting in improved breathing.

Placement

Repeat the setup for Variation 1, but use one bolster placed under the very bottom of the buttocks.

What to Do

As you extend both legs to the right hand, rotate the belly and navel to the left as the right kidney descends. Come up and adjust. Extend the arms, move the legs to the left shoulder, and rotate the belly and navel to the right. The left kidney descends. Deflate the belly toward the back.

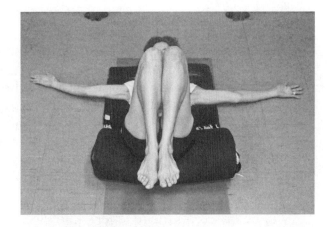

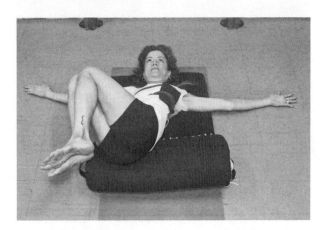

BACK EXTENSIONS

The back extensions are important asanas to offer expansion and vitality. For scoliosis this family of asanas is to be done carefully and with support. Scoliosis, being a three-dimensional pattern, has a very strong influence on the vertebrae, which results in the concavity of the back and overly flexible areas that are destabilized and weak. Although these asanas are extremely important to create the proper energetics for expansion, they need to be addressed conservatively with the support of props. Props provide a passive and beneficial way to perform these asanas, which require a strong back and spine. When done correctly, they offer a feeling of vitality and endurance. Breathing is very important to prevent overexertion and compressions.

Principles in Doing Back Extensions

1. Do not compress the spine.
2. The back of the body serves as a platform for the front when doing back extensions, elongating the anterior spine. In the back extensions done on the floor, the front of the body moves toward the back. The abdominal muscles and asanas strengthen the trunk.
3. The convex ribs are to be more active and faster during the extension. The concave ribs lengthen, and the anterior body restrains the back body from further caving in.
4. There are many ways to prop and belt the torso to provide a compacted and stabilized position for both sides, so during these asanas, the extension should not aggravate the scoliosis. A qualified teacher can find the proper support for your curve.
5. Some cautions: Avoid back extensions during the menstrual period or if you have high blood pressure, glaucoma, extreme fatigue, or spinal fusions (they require a special technique and support), or if you are pregnant. It is important for students to check with an orthopedist to find out what is possible and what is not. Other modifications will be based on the teacher's knowledge of the individual student.

CHATURANGA DANDASANA: FOUR-LIMBED STAFF

Props

Mat, bolster.

Benefits

It strengthens the muscles of the arms (biceps), back, and abdomen. The support of the bolster is an excellent means to experience this strong asana. Even in cases of chiphotic scoliosis, it teaches the proper action for the spine and therefore prepares for the rest of the back extension group of asanas. The muscles hug the bones, and the limbs offer a compact midline position.

Placement

Place a bolster lengthwise on the middle of the mat. Lie face down on the bolster. Bring the hands to the floor next to the chest. Extend both legs, tuck the toes, and extend the heels. The legs are positioned as in tadasana. Look to the front, press the toes and palms into the floor, and attempt to lift both sides of the body parallel to the floor.

What to Do

Anchor the toes, extend the legs evenly, move the tailbone in, lift the ribs away from the pelvis, and move the elbows in, mainly on the convex side. Press down harder with the hand of the concave side, and bring the front to fill and support the back. Look to the front, rest, and release the front of the body on the bolster.

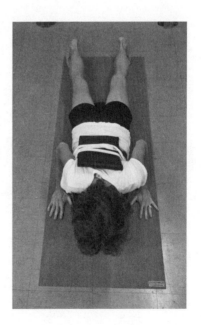

URDHVA MUKHA SVANASANA: UPWARD-FACING DOG

Props

Mat, bolster.

Benefits

Extends both sides and the front of the spine, strengthens the spine, and removes muscular holdings and discomfort caused by the overworked and underworked muscles.

Placement

Place a bolster on the middle of the mat, with blocks on either side if you need them. Lie face down on the bolster. Separate the legs hip-width apart. Press the hands, and tilt the torso up; the spine moves in from the lift. With the hand at the convex ribs, adjust the ribs in toward the spine. Press the hands on the floor or use two blocks if necessary. Press the hand of the concave side to lift and spread the ribs away from the spine. The concave side is to be supported by the front. The front restrains the back from caving further in. Lift both sides of the chest up, reach from the crown of the head, and look up from your chest toward the convex side.

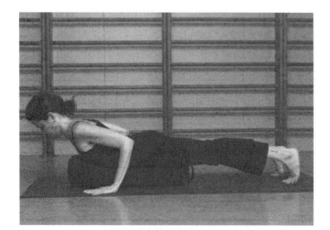 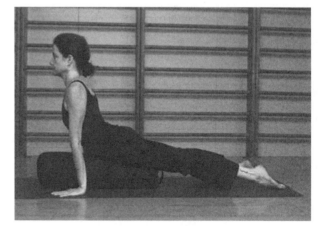

DHANURASANA: BOW POSE

Props

Mat, blankets, belt.

Benefits

The action of the limbs extends the spine and helps the proper adjustment for each side. It promotes anterior extension of the spine and tones the abdominal organs.

Placement

Fold one or two blankets in half to support the waist. Place them on the middle of the mat. Lie down with the waist supported by the blankets. Extend the legs and arms. Lift one leg at a time to elongate that side; do it an extra time on the concave side. Place the arms next to the body with the palms facing up. Extend the arms to move the shoulders down. Press the middle of the buttocks down (sacrum), and bend both legs simultaneously. Grasp both ankles with both hands instead of one at a time. In scoliosis, the limbs move in different patterns; be aware of that and synchronize the movement. If you cannot hold the feet, take two belts and loop each one on the ankle. Pull and lift the legs up; the legs are hip-width apart. With the outer knees in, move the feet toward the ceiling. Take a quick look back, or ask your teacher to view the symmetry of your feet. The pulling of the legs will provide the extension of the arms. Lift the chest and look up. Come out of the pose by releasing the hands and legs.

Note

Do not press the lower back to lift the limbs. Use the limbs and core muscles to lift up.

Note

Before attempting to pick up both legs and lift, break down with one leg at a time to understand the difference between both sides, then complete the asana with both legs lifting.

What to Do

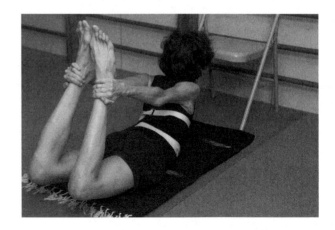

As you grasp the legs, move the convex ribs and shoulder blade in and the concave front ribs back to support the back ribs. One side moves forward as the other creates resistance by moving the contents of the front backward. A way to bring symmetry to the feet is to have the big toes touch for a second. Press the middle layer of the buttocks down, and pull and lift the legs up. Press the shinbone toward the hands, and lift the chest. Add an extra push on the concave side to create space. Roll the shoulders back as you move the convex rib in and the concave rib out. Look up fluidly with both eyes. Come down.

SALABHASANA: LOCUST POSE

Props

Mat, two blankets, two blocks and belt.

Benefits

Tones and strengthens the back muscles (extensors), relieves mild lower back pain.

Placement

Lie face down on a bolster. Take the two blocks and place them next to the outer hips. Place the arms next to the body with the palms of the hands facing down. Extend the arms and legs, and lift the chest off the floor. Look forward and up and lift the chest as you press the middle of the pubic bone down.

If the torso is rolling to one side because of the pull of your curve, come out and place a second bolster adjacent to the first one, wrapped with a belt so they do not come apart. In this case, the blocks might not work, so use the hands to press the bolster instead.

What to Do

Press both hands on the support, and bring the shoulders away from the ears and the shoulder blades in. Extend the limbs as you lift the head, neck, chest, and legs. Maintain the pressure from your hands. Do not press the spine to lift the limbs.

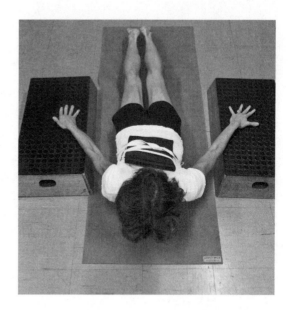

Note

A small pad can be used to support the ventral prominence of the ribs and the concave areas as well. As you get acquainted to your curve you will be able to best judge how to support it.

For lumbar curves, further extend the legs of the curved side, as if someone is pulling your foot out, and move the spine in.

Move both legs simultaneously to the side of the curve. To maintain the legs firm and together, wrap a belt around the middle of the shin bone. Use blocks for the hands.

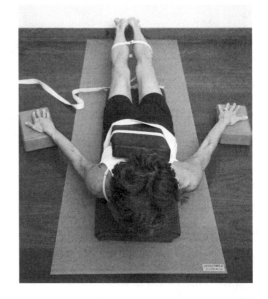

USTRASANA: CAMEL POSE

Props

Wall, mat, bolster, blankets, blocks, chair.

Benefits

This pose creates spinal and pelvic extension, releases the shoulders from elevating, strengthens and tones the back, and inhibits the convexities.

Placement

Fold a mat in half and place a chair between the mat and a wall. Fold a blanket and cover the mat.

Facing the chair, kneel down with the legs hip-width apart and the feet pointing back; the lower legs are parallel. Observe if one leg is rolling out. The thighs are perpendicular to the floor. Place the bolster horizontally between the chair and the pelvis, place the blocks to the outsides of the feet. The pubic bone should be in contact with the bolster. Holding the sides of the chair, pull the hands and lift the chest; lean back and release one hand at a time and move them to the top of the blocks or bolster. If this is not possible, add more height. As the head extends back, lift the chest, placing more emphasis on the convex side.

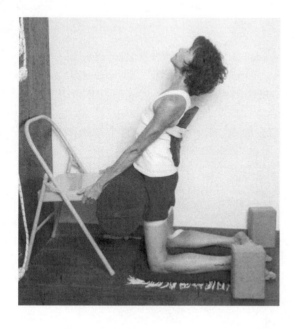
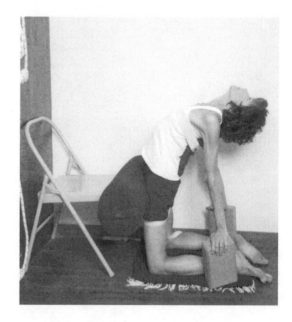

What to Do

Lengthen the shins and press them down as the feet extend. Pull the hamstrings up toward the buttock bone as the shins push down, to add extra pressure on the concave side and to lift the ribs up. Press the right hand and bring the convex ribs in and toward the wall. Push with the left hand and lift the concave side. Lengthen the tail bone and lift the pubic bone toward the bolster. Lift the top of the sacrum up as the back elongates. Bring the hands to the waist and maintain the lift of the chest, releasing each hand one at a time onto the blocks. Add more height as necessary.

Note

Do not push or compress the spine. This is a lift and a back elongation.

Inversions

Inversions are a very important group of asanas. They are also called viparita sthiti. They are medicines for the nervous, endocrine, and immune and fluid systems. An asana practice that includes inversions creates homeostasis, because it brings balance to the autonomic nervous system (sympathetic, parasympathetic); it reduces nervous conditions, as the brain and the head glands receive proper blood supply; it reduces physical and immune fatigue, as the neck glands receive proper blood supply (the thyroid gland regulates cellular metabolism, and the thymus serves as the primary organ of the lymphatic system); and it provides the lungs with a fresh supply of blood. The inversions need to be modified for the asymmetric load of weight produced by the scoliotic spine, but they should not be missed. (For the traditional asanas and sequence, please see *Light on Yoga* by B. K. S. Iyengar.)

Practice under the guidance of a teacher, especially when hanging from the ropes, because the ropes must be tightened properly to avoid accidents. An experienced teacher will show you how to get in the ropes and how to prop for your individual curve.

Caution

Inversions are contraindicated during the menstrual period or if you have neck problems, glaucoma, or high blood pressure.

SALAMBA SIRSASANA: SUPPORTED HEADSTAND

This is considered the most important of the asanas and is referred by the ancient books as the king of the asanas. The preparations for sirsasana came from previous postures such as adho mukha virasana, adho mukha svanasana, uttanasana, and prasarita padottanasana—all are done with support for the head. This asana will teach you how to receive the benefits from the beginning stages of being upside down. Sirsasana with ropes provides the upside-down effects with traction because you are able to hang. If you are unable to use the ropes for the inversions, combine the postures mentioned previously with support for the head (see chapter 5).

The traction offered by the rope in this upside-down position is very satisfying for scoliosis. The gravitational pull is reversed, increasing the sense of internal space on the organic body; the length of the asymmetric load is on the extensors, as the vertebrae and ribs receive the gravitational message to decompress and derotate. It works with the vestibular nerves located inside the inner ears that informs the body of its position and space and how to balance through proprioception. Overall, it offers freedom from the asymmetric shape.

The downside of hanging in ropes for a long time can result in instability and ligament laxity. To resolve this, do not simply collapse the weight because it will fall into the scoliosis. The mind and the body must be alert, so they can adjust the pressure caused by the organs when pushing the bones and when stabilizing the joints that are loose from the action of the muscles. The organic suspension offered by inversions act as an internal traction for the spine and the release of muscular holdings caused by the asymmetry. Even when hanging from the ropes, the feet and toes reach up and spread, as in the first standing asana, tadasana. Arms remain active to adjust the ribs and the shoulders.

Note

Avoid rope sirsasana if you have sacrum pain; the pressure of the rope is intense and it will only aggravate the pain. Also, do not attempt this posture during the menstrual period, or if you have neck problems, glaucoma, high blood pressure, or if you are a beginner student with a fused spine. Get your physician's permission and learn from a senior teacher to ensure the best and safest techniques with the proper support.

If you do not have ropes on the wall, a pelvic swing can be purchased from yoga props suppliers; see Resources.

ROPE SALAMBA SIRSASANA

Props

Ropes on the wall or ceiling, blankets, wooden plank, block. Use two tall ropes, each one hooked from the upper rings. The third rope is tied in between. Have a teacher or an assistant help in setting up.

Benefits

Elongation of the spine.

Placement

Fold two blankets and place them on either side of the ropes. Adjust the ropes, so they are positioned behind you, on the middle of the sacrum. Maintain this position, hold the side ropes, and walk your feet up to a right angle. Now, your teacher or assistant will place an extra blanket and then a wooden plank on top of your legs (in front of the thighs). The assistant will help you in releasing your body down slowly and in extending both legs straight up. A block can be placed between the heels to increase the lift from the inner legs and spine. You will end up in an inverted position, with the legs extended, and the hands holding the plank.

What to Do

Lengthen the feet and lift the inner legs, hold the plank from underneath with the fingers facing front as the shoulder blades move in and up, and maintain the lift of the legs. The tailbone and abdomen move in, and the navel lifts. Compact the convex ribs from the activation of the hands and the arms as the concave side leg lengthens. Let gravity act on the concave side as the leg reaches up toward the ceiling. Ask your teacher or assistant to help you to come out of the posture. Rest in Adho Mukha Virasana (Chapter 4—prone postures). Let the gravity act on the concave and short side.

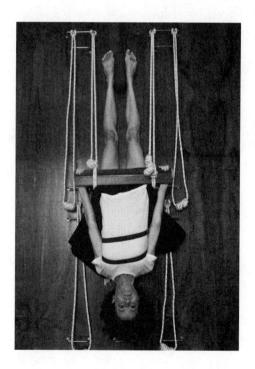

Variation 1: With Support

Props

One or two bolsters, or three to four blankets, wooden wedge, block, belt. Repeat the variation mentioned previously and let the head be supported. Soften the eyes.

Benefits

The support for the head gives proprioception of the spine and creates a soothing condition and feeling of deep rest.

Placement

Repeat the variation above with the additional support for the head. The support should not be too tight as it will compress the spine; the head touches the support without pressing on it. Support the crown of the head with the proper height for you. Once in the position, hold each elbow with the opposite hand.

What To Do

Lift both the inner and outer edges of the legs, and as you hold the elbows bring the shoulders away from the ears and move the shoulder blades in toward the ribs. Bring the convex side in, lift the concave side leg up, and spread the ribs. Work with the curves while upside down. Ask for help before coming out of the posture, then rest in adho mukha virasana.

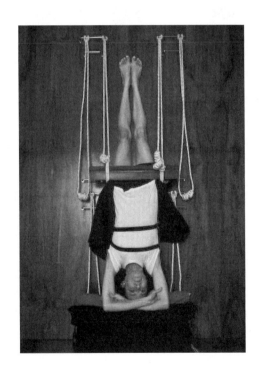

Caution

Do not look to the side. It will cause cervical spine problems.

Variation 2: Boxed Salamba Sirsasana

This variation is not for the beginner student.

Props

Halasana box, mat, blanket, pads, wall.

Benefits

The independent upside-down position is not ideal for scoliosis because it brings compression. You need the aid of a teacher if you are going to be able to do it. The benefits of being upside down have already been mentioned, as well as the cautions. Carefully consider both. Inversions are just another option in case one decides to experience the supervised independence of being upside down for a small amount of time.

Placement

Place the box on the wall, with the open end facing you. Have two or more pads on the sides of it to offer a compacted position mainly to the convex side. Fold a blanket lengthwise in three so it will look like a tube. The height of the blanket will vary for each person. If the shoulders are collapsing this means that the height of the blankets has to be increased. Kneel down and place the forearms inside the box, with the elbows a shoulder width apart and the inner upper arms parallel. Interlock all the fingers, with the tips of the thumbs touching (not crossed). The interlock creates a cup. The weight will be in the forearms. Release the crown of the head on the blanket; lift and widen the shoulders as the wrists and forearms press and the box creates a resistance for your forearms. Tuck the toes under, and slowly straighten the legs and lift the hips. Walk the feet toward the shoulders. Bend both legs in, and lift both legs to the wall. Place both heels on the wall.

What to Do

As you press the forearms, spread the shoulder and outer elbows against the box and lift the legs up. Lift the concave leg further up. Do not stay in this position long if you feel strain. Try decentralizing the legs to bring asymmetric spine stability.

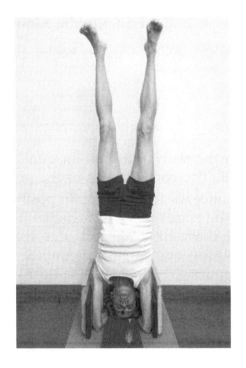

ROPE ADHO MUKHA VIRASANA: DOWNWARD-FACING HERO POSE

Props

Blanket, wooden plank, rope, wall.

Benefits

Facing the wall has a soothing quality as the sensory organs are withdrawing from external stimuli. The compactness of the position, along with the gravitational pull, releases the spine, and the plank helps the shoulders to stabilize and the chest to open. It offers proprioception to the back body, and addresses correction for the ribs.

Placement

Stand behind the ropes with the back on the wall. Hold the bottom of the rope where you will be sitting, and move it over to your head and down to the top of your thighs, as if you are putting on a shirt. Shift your body weight to the front so your feet will come off the floor. Bend both legs, move the shinbones to the wall, and continue lowering your body; you will end with your head toward the floor and your legs bent on the wall with the rope supporting the upper legs. Have an assistant place a wooden plank behind your back as you hook your arms around it. This position resembles how a bat sleeps.

What To Do

Press the shin bone on the wall, coil the shoulders and lift them up. Bring both sides of the waist back. To come out of the posture ask for help, then immediately rest in adho mukha virasana.

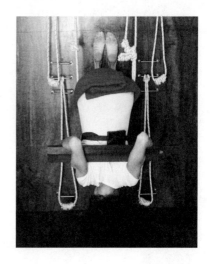

ROPE PARSVA ADHO MUKHA VIRASANA: DOWNWARD-FACING HERO TO THE SIDE

Following the pose mentioned previously, have a teacher or an assistant release the wooden plank from your back. Release the arms, stabilize the right hand, and walk with the left finger tips under the right arm as the left ribs spread out. If this is the concave side, elongate the left hand a little farther. Return to the center. Stabilize the left hand and walk with the right fingertips under the left arm. The head is centered in this variation. Repeat the variation and let the head follow the movement of the hand to create a twisted action.

Benefits

The twisted movement helps the counter rotation of the curves and brings mobility to the organs. It also offers spinal elongation.

What To Do

As the right hand presses down, move the left hand under and revolve and broaden the left ribs toward the right side. As the left hand stabilizes, work the right hand under and revolve with the right ribs. For right thoracic scoliosis, bring the ribs in. Ask for help to come out of the position (slowly), and rest in adho mukha virasana.

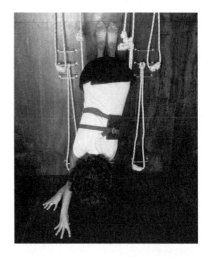

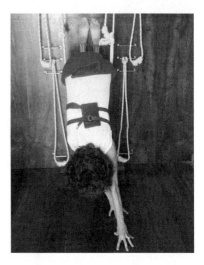

CHAIR SALAMBA SARVANGASANA: CHAIR SHOULDERSTAND

Sarvangasana is considered the queen of the asanas. Similar to salamba sirsasana, this asana is to be learned and practiced under the guidance of a teacher, so the proper support is offered. Scoliosis requires an outside professional eye to help with one's alignment, because our proprioception is organized within the asymmetry (distortion). Learning how to use the props, mainly in inversions, requires repetition and safety.

Props

Two mats, wall, one chair, three blankets or bolster, extra pads, small roll.

Note

If the cervical spine reverses the curve, place a roll under the neck or add more height.

Placement

Place the back of the chair a couple of inches away from the wall and place a bolster or two rectangular (lengthwise) folded blankets on the floor. Place a symmetrically folded mat on the edge of the chair seat to create support and traction for the sacral spine. Sit on the side of the chair, then turn to face the back of the chair and place one leg at a time over it. Both legs will be hooked over the back of the chair. Move the back body to the blankets or bolster; the shoulders will be on the blankets, and the neck and the head will be on the floor. The waist is on the seat of the chair. Hold the chair with the hands, and stretch the legs so the heels are on the wall and the back of the legs rest on the back of the chair. Note that for lumbar scoliosis the pelvis will tilt and rotate to one side. Insert a pad on the opposite side, between the outer hip and the chair, to bring evenness.

What to Do

Hold the chair, roll and align the shoulders, and lift the middle of the chest. Activate the arms and bring the convex ribs in and the concave ribs out. Lift the middle of the chest and lengthen both legs. Keep holding the chair, lifting the body, and adjusting the position of the ribs. The convex ribs move toward the ceiling, and the front ribs of the concave side move back to fill the back ribs. Do not stay in this posture too long; it is challenging and it can cause the body to collapse on the chair.

Avoid dropping the weight to the chair.

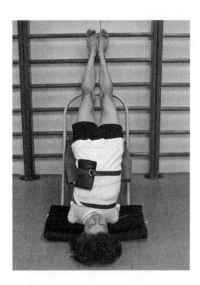

Variation

Follow the variation above and descentralize the legs. Use an additional mat for the buttocks as necessary. This posture offers stability as it decreases the wobbling feeling when the legs are together. It spreads the front, the back, and the sides of the trunk.

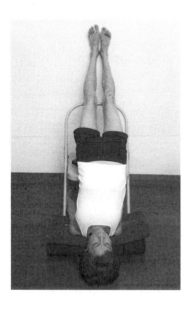
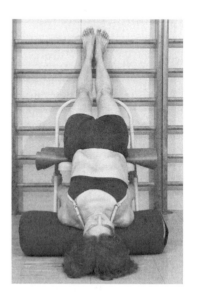

HALASANA: PLOW POSE

Props

Mat, two chairs, two or three blankets or bolster.

Benefits

Improves breathing on the concave side.

Placement

From the chair on sarvangasana, bring both legs to the second chair. Hold the back with both hands with fingers facing up. With your hand, push the convex ribs in and fill the concave ribs from the front. Lift both sides of the trunk. To come out, bend the legs and roll them down.

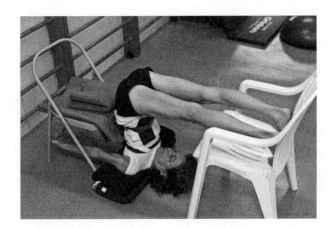

Restorative Savasana: Witnessing and Feeling the Breath

Medical research on idiopathic scoliosis has linked the pathology to the insufficient production of the hormone melatonin, which affects the asymmetric growth of the vertebrae. Melatonin is produced by the pineal gland during the night, in conditions of darkness. During a yoga class or personal practice, the restorative postures, savasana (resting pose), and pranayama (breathing practices) can be done with the room lights dim or with the eyes covered with a cloth or eye mask. The darkness provides the experience of deep organic rest; as the organs rest, the nerves rest and awareness of the breath increases, which brings a state of homeostasis to the nervous system. Doing these practices in semidarkness has a different effect than doing them during daylight. These biochemical changes, which also come from the combination and proper sequence of asanas, act as medicine for the various body systems: nervous, endocrine, musculoskeletal, organic, respiratory, and circulatory.

The restorative postures can be done any time; and savasana, the final rest, is not to be skipped after the asana practice. The breathing practices (pranayama), as the asanas, are to be learned under the assistance of a teacher and modified accordingly for the individual. The breath is the bridge between mind and body, and a very powerful tool that can also harm when not done correctly. It needs to be addressed with sensitivity and intelligence.

The postures below are modified. Please refer to *Light on Pranayama* and *Light on Yoga*, by B. K. S. Iyengar, for the traditional postures and cautions.

SAVASANA

Sava means corpse and *asana* means posture. It involves surrendering of the efforts and actions to the fruit of those efforts and actions. This deep concept of surrender of the mind makes this asana a most challenging one. When we lie down with asymmetries, the mind is constantly tracking the unevenness and trying to self-correct and to find contentment. It raises anxieties and frustrations. To bring the mind to a state of equanimity, there must be the proper support that will increase the height, volume, and width of the chest; stability; and the feeling of inner space created from the support. In Patanjali's *Yoga Sutra*, the second chapter called "Sadhana Pada" describes the eight limbs to achieve yoga (union). The second limb is called nyama, and it has five rules for individual discipline. The last one is called *isvara pranidhana*, which reflects on a profound surrendering to the divine, which means giving over our mind to a higher intelligence and trusting it. (Please view *Light On the Yoga Sutras of Patanjali* with translation by B. K. S. Iyengar).

Savasana is the best asana for studying, feeling, and witnessing yourself; it will show you every minute asymmetry in your body. It is important to find the proper support you need to help the body be as stable and organized toward symmetry as possible to then completely surrender from the actions or attempts to change.

Suggestions

1. Before lying down, make sure that all the props are nearby and organized. Place your mat in a place that has enough space, so your arms and legs can be free. The nervous system cannot rest if the limbs are not at ease. Remove eyeglasses and accessories such as your wristwatch and jewels. Turn off the phones, beepers, etc.

2. When you lie down for savasana, have a teacher help set up the props for proper alignment. This is to be taught and learned.

3. In savasana, the chest is to be elevated, so the diameter of the lungs can open. The concave areas and empty places that do not release to the floor should be supported with props. The body must be totally supported to release to gravity.

4. Center the blankets or bolster evenly on the mat. There are specific yoga mats that have geometric straight lines that give a central reference to the body. Sit on the center of the mat and have a bolster or folded rectangular blankets a couple of inches away, so when you lie down, the floating ribs (T11, T12) will touch the bolster and not your lumbar spine. Roll each vertebra slowly to the bolster and observe where the deviations occur. Have both legs folded with the sole of the feet on the floor. Press the feet and lift the buttock up, and manually scoop the buttocks toward the feet. Hold the back of the head with both hands and gently pull it away from the feet. This is a micro traction.

5. Extend one leg at a time. Notice which leg you tend to use to initiate the movement and shift to the opposite one.
6. The back of the pelvis, the back of the heels, and both legs should move away from the head.
7. Both legs, when extended down, rotate from the big toes to the small toes, as the groin and the pelvic organs soften. The release of the legs is gradual and, with attention, the root of the legs slowly turns and releases out on the hip socket, so there is a connection between the acetabulum of the hip and the head of the femur. The tendency is to lose that connection when there is too much mobility in the ligaments of one side. The organization of the body on the floor is reproduced in standing. Think of the legs as columns.
8. The same applies to the arms. The arms turn out from the thumb to the little finger; there must be a space in the armpit so the side portion of the lungs can find freedom, especially on the retracted side.
9. The shoulders move away from the head, and the lateral angle of the shoulder blades move in and down. With the opposite hand, adjust the shoulder blade on the convex side. Move it in and down.
10. The back of the head is centered. Be aware of tilts because it will affect one's proprioception of center. The nose is aligned with the center of the lips, chest bone (sternum), navel, and center of the pubic bone. The cervical spine, top of shoulder blades, and thoracic spine are in contact with the support. Have a folded blanket or a pad for the head, and if there is cervical curve reversal (the chinbone moves down and the throat closes), roll the edge of a blanket under the cervical spine.
11. The tongue rests and is centered on the floor of the mouth.
12. If one side of the chest is closed, take a wooden plank (with the thin edge up) or fold a blanket and place it under the middle of the chest (in the area of the heart). Place small foam pads or wooden wedges under the convex side of the outer shoulder blade to lift the spine and chest. Place small pads under the concave ribs, and wooden wedges under the outer edges of the pelvis as it tends to rotate front (lumbar curve). The pads and the wedges will make the shoulders, ribs, and pelvis even.
13. Weights are one of my favorite props; they are used to ground the areas that lift from gravity. These suspended and retracted areas are caused by the spinal rotation, and create a pull on the organs and nerves. Weights can be used for different areas and with different loads. It is often used in the final savasana in the root of the upper thighs, on the center of sacrum in prone savasana, in the space between the upper arm and top of the chest (upper armpit), and light a weight can be placed on the top of the convexities, as well as for the hands and forehead (forebrain). As the bones and joints receive the weight, the contact to the ground is enhanced, creating a feeling of stability, organization, and deep rest. It is a surrendering from the alertness of the asymmetric nerves and mind.
14. To come out of savasana, gradually open the eyes and let the gaze be receptive, bend one leg at a time, roll to the right side, and cradle the head with a blanket as you rest in this fetal position. Use the hands to press the floor, and with the gaze and head down, roll the spine up. The head and the eyes will be last to come to vertical.

Note

The correct way to roll is to the right to avoid pressure on the heart. However, with scoliosis, sometimes it is important to offer both sides a chance to move. Mainly, if the curve is on the right side, it is important to roll to the left.

The Skin

In the womb, as the spine is developing, the back body (ectoderm) gives rise to the epidermis of the skin, the neural tube, the central nervous system, and the peripheral nerves. The skin is an outgrowth of the nervous system; as the skin relaxes, the brain relaxes. Think of the skin as an organ that directs and guides the nervous system. The skin of the forehead descends toward the facial bones; the skin of the neck lengthens on the right and left sides; and the skin of the chest spreads to the right and left sides. The skin of the upper arms rolls from inside out, inducing an external rotation of the arms (head of humerus), with the palms facing up (supination). The top of the chest is like two windows that open. The skin of the top shoulders rolls down toward the back like a waterfall. The skin of the buttocks rolls and scoops down toward the feet. The skin of the whole body breathes. In savasana, the skin, the bones, the muscles, and the organs release to gravity.

The Ears

The head pivots in the space between the ears (inner ear). Both ears are aligned and receptive. Observe if one ear is moving down toward the shoulder and adjust accordingly.

The Eyes

Both eyes are closed but they can look inside of the heart. They can also gravitate back toward the back of the head. Observe if both eyes are evenly released.

The Nose

The nose is a reference for the midline of the face, and the first entrance of the breath. Observe both nostrils and how the breath flows on both sides.

The Mouth

The tongue rests on the floor of the mouth, not tilting to the right or left. Rest the back of the tongue, where it is often lifted and apt to cause tension. The lips are slightly open.

Caution

In case of lower back pain, suspend the legs over a chair (chair savasana, see discussion later). Place a bolster or pillow under the knees. Spread the legs (decentralize). When prone (lying on the back), the toes touch and the heels spread (pigeon toes).

Suggestions for Props

- Belts offer extra feedback to the shoulder blades, ribs, and upper and lower legs to prevent unwanted rotations. Get a helper to assist you in placing the belts, and place them loosely so as not to constrain the breath. Contain the frame of the body by looping a small belt around the big toes, not too tight, and another one on the top of the legs. The belts are to be used only when needed, and according to the individual alignment and need in a more active savasana. Alternate the metal part and end of the belts, so when using several belts, it does not affect and influence the flow of the skin.
- For the thoracic spine, two blocks vertically placed on either side of the spine support and open both sides of the chest. The back of the head is supported with a third block (same height as the others). The inner heels, inner calves, and upper legs can be wrapped with belts. The contained position offered by the blocks offers a midline and core orientation.
- Bolsters might not be for everyone. The round, soft bolsters tend to invite unevenness; they allow the body to roll to one side. They can also be uncomfortable for small people and those with lower back issues. The best bolsters for scoliosis are the rectangular, firm ones that offer stability for both sides. Bolsters placed next to either side of the body offer a sense of compactness. Two bolsters are used for the restorative asanas in case of difficulty in lying down.
- Blankets are excellent to support the asymmetric spine and the appendicular skeleton (limbs, pelvic, and shoulder girdles). To avoid lower back compression and pain, a rolled blanket under the knees is a simple and effective solution. For the spine, I like using two or three folded lengthwise—not narrow, but wide—so both sides of the back spread and feel supported. An extra blanket can be folded horizontally under the middle of the chest to lift and broaden the cardiac spine to support the back of the heart and lungs.
- Wedges or pads compensate for the unevenness of the shoulders and hips (shoulder and pelvic girdles). For right thoracic scoliosis, or a combination of right and left lumbar, where the right shoulder lifts away from the mat, place a pad under the opposite shoulder. The same applies for the pelvis. This is one way to create evenness.

The belt, in general, offers a sense of cohesion and direction for the skin, and when placed on the top of the legs (femoral joint), it prevents the classic asymmetric leg rolling during the supine position.

The following are a few restorative asanas that create the awareness for deep rest and breathing. They create the frame for expansion, elongations, and relaxation. It is difficult to lie or sit for a long period of time and concentrate on the breath, so it is important to practice specific asanas before attempting to deeply rest and breathe. Under the guidance of a teacher, a proper sequence is created to further prepare the asymmetric body to breathe deeply.

My teacher, B. K. S. Iyengar, said that compression leads to deformity. He gave us his brilliant system to uncover the veil of distortions and compressions through the practice of asanas, and the use of various props to provide extension and bring space to the compressive areas.

SUPTA VIRASANA: RECLINED HERO

Props

Mat, one or two bolsters, blankets, wooden plank, wooden wedges, pads, two blocks.

Benefits

Lengthen the hip flexors (iliopsoas) and the abdominal organs and allow the torso to move away from the hips. This is a very important action for scoliosis, especially on the concave side. The abdominal organs recede toward the spine. It helps digestion, and relieves fatigue. This is not a very easy posture for some, but once learned, it can offer amazing benefits to the digestive and nervous systems.

Placement

Place a bolster across the middle of the mat and sit on a block in virasana, with the back to the bolster. Lean back, so that both sides of the upper ribs will face the ceiling and simultaneously curve over the bolster. The bolster is under the center of the shoulder blades. The shoulders roll down and the back of the head rests on a second foam block.

What to Do

Move the outer shoulder blades in and rotate the upper arms with the palm of the hands facing up. Move the convex ribs in, and lengthen the concave side by moving the legs away from the trunk, yet firm the outer hips. Lengthen the tailbone and sacrum away from the lumbar, as the pubic bone lifts up and the abdomen moves back. Move the shoulders away from the ears and spread the chest. To come out, walk with both hands toward the legs, press the hands on the floor, and lift both sides of the trunk. Release the block and stretch one leg at a time in dandasana (staff).

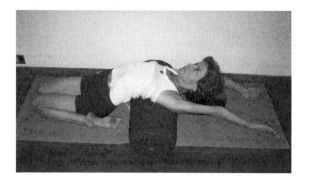

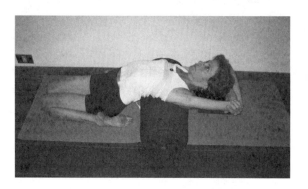

Caution

In case of lower back pain, or in the reclined position, it is not possible. See the following variation.

Variation 1: With a Chair

Props

Mat, wall, chair, bolster, blocks, blankets.

Placement

Place a mat on the wall (vertical). A chair against the wall, one block a couple of inches away from the chair, one bolster lengthwise reclined in between the space of the block and the chair, a pranayama pillow or wooden plank next to the bolster.

Sit on the block in virasana and recline back on the bolster. Move the chest away from the bolster and place the wooden plank or pillow under the middle of the chest. Both sides of the plank or the pillow are centered in relation to the back. Let the hands rest on the sides with the support of blocks. To come out, press both hands on the blocks, look up, lift the chest, and sit in virasana. Stretch both legs at a time in dandasana (staff).

Use an additional bolster or blankets to increase the support for the back. Make sure that the bolsters are centered.

Note

To firm the back of the bolster, use a third block.

Caution

Do not collapse the chest; tilt the torso.

SUPTA BADDHA KONASANA: RECLINED BOUND

Props

Mat, one or two bolsters, belts, blankets, wooden plank, wooden wedges, pads.

Benefits

Softens the groin, lengthens the pelvic and abdominal organs, and opens the lungs and chest.

Placement

Place the bolster in the middle of the mat, with the plank on top. Sit in baddha konasana. If you need to secure the feet from sliding, open a belt and place it under your feet, over the ankles and the thighs, and around the center of the sacrum. Fasten the belt, tighten it, and draw the heels toward the perineum. Lean back, so the bottom edge of the bolster touches the floating ribs, not the lower back, and lower the trunk on the bolster. The wooden plank is under the middle of the chest, and the head and neck are supported by a blanket. The arms rotate and the palms rest facing the ceiling. Next, lengthen the arms over the head and fold the elbows. Hold the elbows with the opposing hand. To come up, fold the legs and release the strap and blanket, press both hands down, and lift up by moving the upper chest in and looking up.

In case of lower back pain, come up by gazing at the navel and pressing the hands. Do it from a rolling action.

Note

To support the thighs, fold the blanket lengthwise and wrap it in front of the ankles, with its end on the outer hips.

Increase the height of the bolster in case of tightness; add a vertical lengthwise-folded blanket on the top of the bolster, or another bolster. But be aware not to compress the lumbar spine. The bolsters touch the junction between the last thoracic vertebra (T12) and the first lumbar (L1).

What to Do

Release the inside of the legs to the knees as the outer hips firm. From the contact of both feet, correct the extra rolling in the pelvis by pressing one foot more than the other. Scoop the buttocks away from the lumbar spine, and lengthen the tailbone toward the feet, lift the pubic bone up, and soften the belly toward the spine. Lengthen both sides of the waist, focusing on the concave side. Move the ribs away from the hips as you pull the elbows over the head. Roll the shoulders down and pull with the plank further in with your hands to bring the shoulder blade on the convex side in. As you hold your elbows, offer an extra pull on the concave side and compact the convex ribs in. Release the elbows and the arms, and rest with the arms alongside of the body before coming up.

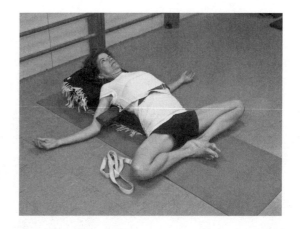

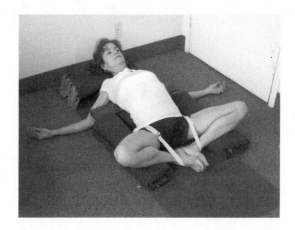

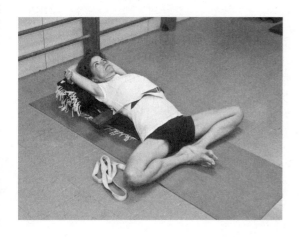

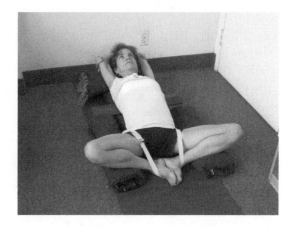

SUPTA SWASTIKASANA: RECLINED AUSPICIOUS POSE

Repeat the preceding variation. This position brings the head of the femur in, and it offers a sense of containment for the abdominal organs. For some, it will be a challenging position, mainly when the curve is on the lumbar spine. In this case, increase the height of the support for the back, and if this is not helpful, stay in supta baddha konasana.

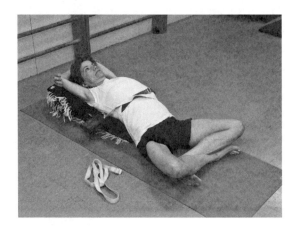

SUPTA TADASANA: RECLINED MOUNTAIN POSTURE

Props

Mat, blanket, three blocks, three belts for the legs, pads, wooden wedges.

Benefit

It promotes midline orientation and rest.

Placement

Fold a blanket in quarters and place it in the middle of the mat. Sit in dandasana, with the feet to the wall, and place the blocks in three areas: between the inner heels, between the calves, and between the upper groins. The belts will tie each segment. They should counter each other and offer the proper alignment for the skin. Lie down in the center and adjust the posture: the back of the pelvis and the back of the heels away from the head. Roll the shoulders and upper arms back. Roll the thumb toward the floor. If a shoulder lifts, place pads under the opposite shoulder; do the same for the pelvis.

Note

The face releases toward the back of the skull, and the eyes toward the feet. The back of the head is centered. With an upper thoracic or cervical curve, the head will tilt. To align the head, bring the tip of the nose to the center of the lips (clavicle notch) and center of the chest (sternum). Place two small rolls next to each side of the neck to prevent the head from rolling to one side.

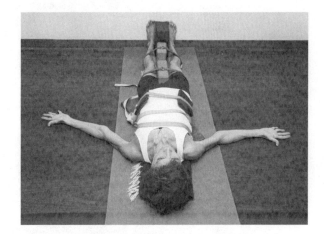

Variation 1: With Weights

Props

Mat, blanket, wedges.

Benefits

The placement of weight on the joints enhances proprioception. As the body feels weighted, the nervous system releases its ongoing control and alertness. It is nice to place sandbags on the belly to bring the organs back toward the nerves and spine. There are many possibilities to explore the placement of the different weights. The wedges help prevent pelvic and shoulder rotation and bring evenness to both sides.

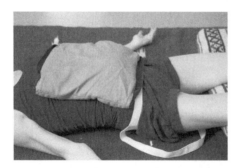
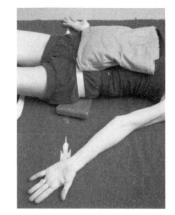
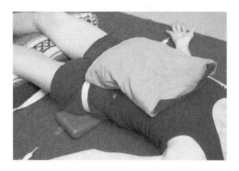
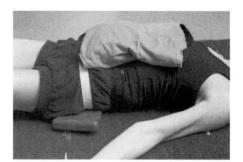

SETU BANDHA SARVANGASANA: BRIDGE POSE

This is a very important asana that lengthens the front of the spine and opens the chest. One side of the scoliosis is overly extended and the opposite is tight. The extension of the legs results in the activation of the deeper muscles (iliopsoas major), core stabilization, and midline orientation. The blocks are used to induce the tailbone to move in and to let the front body release toward the back. The ribs separate from the pelvis, mainly on the short side. It tones both sides of the paraspinal muscles (extensors) and the spine as it draws in. The pose opens the lungs, heart, and chest and generates vitality and joy.

SETU BANDHA

Variation 1

Props

Wall, mat, four bolsters, pads, two or more blankets.

Note

If you do not have all the props, there are other means to support the feet and the spine. In this photo, I am using boxes for this exercise. We need to work with what we have and use the environment as an option.

Placement

Place two stacked horizontal bolsters on the floor against a wall to support the feet, two stacked lengthwise (vertical) bolsters one-and-a-half feet away from the wall to support the spine, and two to three folded blankets to support the head. Sit on the bolsters closer to the wall, place a strap on the top of the thighs, and lean back on the bolsters with the shoulders and back of the head on the floor. Place the legs on the wall and extend the legs with the feet on the wall. Roll the shoulders back to the upper arms and let the arms rest on the floor. To come out, bend the legs and place the feet on the floor and slide back until the pelvis and the torso are on the floor. Roll to the right side and come up.

Note

The props here are very high; in case of disc injuries and hernia, avoid this asana.

What to Do

Press the feet, extend the legs, soften the abdomen, and roll the upper arms and shoulders. The forehead releases toward the chest. Compact the convex ribs in, as you roll the right upper arm out and move the shoulder blade in. Spread the concave ribs out and release.

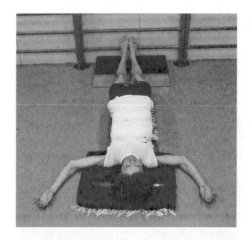

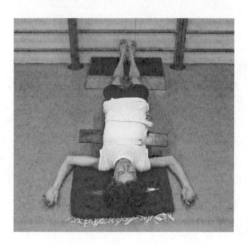

PRONE SAVASANA

Props

Mat, bolster.

Benefits

This is a very simple savasana and easy to set up. It is very relaxing as the organic body is supported and both sides spread.

Placement

Place the bolster toward the front of the mat. Lie on it, with the pubic bone touching the bolster and the legs spread out, rest the forehead on the hands.

What to Do

Extend both legs as you lengthen the feet and move the little toes in line with the outer edges of the mat as both sides of the waist extend and the shoulders roll down. Release the forehead, the eyes, the jaw, and the tongue. Press the elbows slightly down and adjust the sides of your rib cage. Move the convex ribs in, spread the concave ribs, and elongate both sides away from your legs.

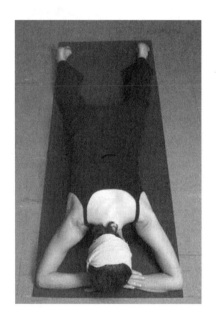

Note

If the body is rolling to one side add an extra bolster underneath your trunk and make sure that both bolsters are centered and supporting both sides.

Variation 1: Prone Savasana

Props

Mat, six or seven blankets, two bolsters.

Benefits

In this pose, the organic body releases to gravity and supports the back, and the back spreads. The parasympathetic branch of the autonomic nervous system predominates in this resting position, as the organs are receiving a fresh supply of blood.

Placement

Place a horizontal bolster on the middle of the mat and lie with your belly on the bolster. As the lower buttock bone rolls down and the legs extend and spread to the sides, be aware if one leg tends to roll further out. Support the concave side of the body from the front with an additional blanket or pads. The head can be supported on a block or with your hands. Follow the directions of the previous variation.

Bend the arms to the side in a cactus position; this will flatten the bulges of the spine and ribs, and spread the chest and sternum. Add two blankets, folded in quarters, to support the anterior portion of the upper arms, so the armpit does not collapse in. Add two bolsters or two folded blankets for the elbows, lower arms, and hands. Make sure the fold is more or less symmetrical. The shoulder blades cut inward. Place a blanket under the forehead so the head is aligned with the spine and the nose is free to breathe.

Use extra blankets if you need them. In case of lumbar pain and compression under the pelvis, fold a blanket in half, and place it between the pubic bone and lower floating rib; this will help the asymmetries of the iliac crest and decompress the lumbar spine. The right and left buttocks descend down away from the lumbar spine. A teacher should check the asymmetries of the shoulders and pelvis, and even them with extra pads or wedges.

The key for scoliosis is to spread the back skin fibers equally, the right to the right and the left to the left. The spine is supported by the front. If one side is rolling more, adjust the support so both sides are properly supported and the nerves can rest.

What to Do

Release the belly to the bolster and extend the legs. Extend each leg back and roll the inner edge to the outer. Bring the convex ribs in and down toward the bolster as the concave ribs spread.

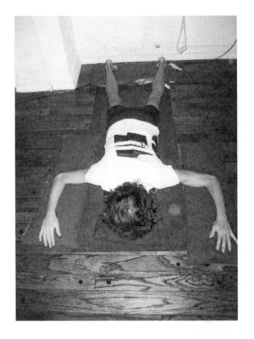

Variation 2: Asymmetric (Akounchanasana)

Props

Mat, bolster, blankets or pillows, pads.

Benefits

This savasana reflects the homolateral ontogenetic pattern that babies do to organize and differentiate the body sides, and that I feel has been skipped with scoliosis. This position extends and differentiates the right and left sides, and helps to release sacroiliac joint compression as the organic body releases toward the opposite side.

Placement

Lie in prone position, with the pelvis resting on a bolster across the mat. Extend both arms in line with the shoulders, with the convex shoulder and leg bent (my major curve is on the right side). The thigh is at a 90-degree angle, with the knee in line with the buttock. Support the knee with an additional blanket or block to prevent it from strain. Extend the leg down and have your teacher or assistant roll a blanket under the ankle, and use additional blankets to support the armpits, the head, and the front of the concave ribs. The head turns toward the bent leg side and both ears are parallel. The arm on the concave side is higher to further elongate and spread the ribs on that side. Place an extra pad under the ventral prominence (front convexity).

What to Do

Firm the convex side in. Release and relax the concave.

When going to the short side, instead of lateral bending (flexion) to that side, spread the ribs out and elongate the arm. Stay longer on this side. As you flex the convex side, extend the convex by lengthening the arm over the head and spreading the ribs to the side.

Note

The principle is to stay longer on the side that provides the extension of the concave (short) side. Moreover, when flexing the leg on the short side, work the left ribs, lift away from the pelvis, and spread to the side away from the spine. For the lumbar curve it is the same principle, the legs will help the spine to move in and the hip down.

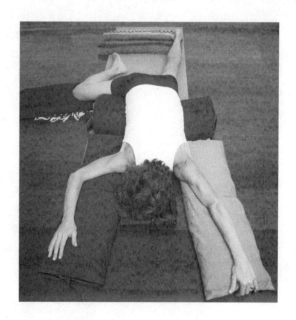

CHAIR SAVASANA

Props

Mat, three blankets, chair, belt, eye mask, sandbag or weight on abdomen to further decrease lumbar contraction.

Placement

Face the chair. Place one folded blanket on the chair seat, another one at the top of the mat for the head to maintain the cervical curve. Place one folded blanket for the pelvis. Place another folded blanket, not too thick, for the lumbar spine.

Sit facing the chair, slide the buttocks toward the chair and lie down. Bend the legs and place the lower legs on the chair seat. The outer buttock bones should cut down toward the floor, so have the knees at a slightly oblique angle to the feet. Use a loose belt to constrain the legs from falling outward. Place the pads under the concave side, and for the shoulders and pelvis.

Place the arms alongside the torso, press both hands down, and move the buttocks toward the chair. Lift your forearms and press both elbows down evenly to move the shoulder blades in and away from the ears. Scoop the buttocks and roll the shoulders back. Without disturbing the position created, hold the head and slightly traction it away from the tailbone.

Very Important

Observe the alignment of the pelvis; if one pelvic half lifts away from the floor, place a thin blanket or pad under the opposite pelvis in line with the femur joint. Use pads or blankets to fill any major concavity. The back must yield to the floor, yet maintain its curve. In case of discomfort because of sacroiliac pain and compression, explore lying on the convex side with the left leg partially bent; you can place a pillow between the legs, and hug a bolster to add dimension and fullness in the front body. Place a blanket under the head. Use an eye mask to bring the awareness inside your breath and enjoy.

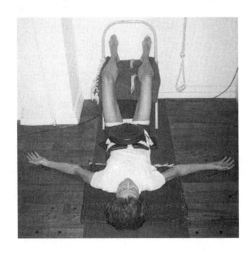

WITNESSING AND FEELING THE BREATH

Life is breath, and breath is movement. Breath underlies function and form. Breath changes the shape of our structure, as it enlivens muscles and tissues. Breath supports the spine and posture as it strengthens the muscles of respiration—the external and internal costal and the diaphragm. Breath enhances our life force and energy.

The diaphragm has its insertion on T12. As soon as we breathe, the spine moves. Posture can be improved by breathing. Automatic breathing is controlled by the brain stem—the reptilian brain; the lack of full breathing affects the physical, organic, and mental layers of the self.

Following the steps of Patanjali's asthanga yoga, pranayama is the limb that follows the asanas. First, we need to align our physical structure to go deeper within. After a strong asana practice, we continue the inner journey from the gross to the subtle. The art of pranayama is a very important and profound subject, and must be taught by your teacher according to your level. Breath is related to our life force, mind, and emotions, and how we live in the world. In yoga, breath is the bridge between mind and body, and it is always done through the nose, unless otherwise instructed. In yogic breathing practice or pranayama, various specialized breathing methods enhance the depth, diameter, and dimensions of the body.

The first stage is to observe the cycles of inhalation and exhalation and the pauses in between. Do not attempt to do these practices without guidance; they can cause harm in the nervous system.

Space and Air

In scoliosis, the notion of space is obscure; the organs feel undifferentiated, compressed, and collapsed because of adhesions that prevent mobility and the flow of the breath. If one side is contracted and closes, the lung and muscles of respiration are compressed, not leaving much space for the breath to flow with ease. Oxygen travels where there is space, not where there is compression. Witnessing the breath opens the possibilities for inner space within the organs and areas that are compressed.

In scoliosis, the breath flows differently on the concave and convex sides. The inhalations can be perceived from the convex side, and less so on the concave. Both sides are to be addressed because of the rotation on the ribs. The main thing is to lift both sides of the chest with the help of props and to adjust both sides of the ribcage. The lobes of the lungs, mainly the upper lobes (slightly above the clavicles), are to spread and receive the air. The external and internal costal muscles, mainly on the concave side, are to lengthen and tone. This retracted side is weak and does not receive the same supply of oxygen, and the side that protrudes the anterior upper chest closes because of the pull of the curve. The result is fatigue, depression, confusion, and organic compression.

One of the prognoses of scoliosis is that its progression will compromise the spinal cord and organs of respiration. Surgery is sometimes necessary to save the lungs and to improve quality of life.

The practice of witnessing and feeling the breath will enhance the awareness and intelligence in areas that are dormant and will prevent further deterioration.

The breath in scoliosis will indicate the asymmetries of ribs, pelvis, shoulders, lungs, and diaphragm of both sides. The breath will indicate where one needs to further open space.

The inhalation cycles can offer great insight about the retracted side and the upper chest. The upper lobes expand when the inhalation is full. This creates volume and a convex shape for the caved shape. The exhalation cycles will decrease the tone of the pulling, leading to a deflation of the convex side. The breath then comes to create symmetry in both sides with long inhalations and long exhalations. Note that the relationship of the breath shifts according to the body's position. In supine postures, there is an upward motion of the convex ribs, which tend to collapse. The inhalation cycle would lift and bring the bulging ribs in.

SUPPORTED SAVASANA

Props

Mat, four blankets, wooden plank, wooden wedges, pads, small cloths.

Benefits

In Savasana, the utilization of extra support is used to improve one's alignment, so the chest and lungs can bloom like a flower while the body can deeply rest. The support under the chest will facilitate breath flow in the chest cavity, where the oxygen first reaches. A feeling of evenness is created from slow breathing.

Bringing awareness to the breath focuses the mind and enhances the intelligence of both sides.

Placement

Fold three blankets in fourths lengthwise or vertically to support the spine. To avoid patterns of rolling from the scoliosis, the fold should not be too narrow. Place a wooden plank toward the back of the mat to support and lift the middle of the chest. Fold a fourth blanket to support the cervical spine, the back, and the head. The number of blankets for the trunk and head will depend on the person's structure.

Sit with the legs bent and the buttocks a couple of inches away from the blanket; adjust the buttocks flesh. Be aware of being in the center. Have a teacher to help, or a mirror. As you lie down, make sure that the floating ribs touch the support, not the lumbar spine (lower back). With the hands, pull the skull away from the buttocks and the buttocks flesh toward the feet. Move the tailbone in. Lengthen one leg at a time away from the head, and gradually let each leg release. Roll the shoulders back; the convex side shoulder rolls more. The wooden wedges are helpful to insert under the convex side protracted shoulder blade. They also lift the chest and align the outer shoulders and pelvis from the rotation (pelvis asymmetry).

Note

The props are helpful accessories to align the shoulders and pelvis for the asymmetric rotations, protractions, and retractions, but most of all, to lift the areas that drop under both sides of the chest, and freeing the lungs to receive your breath.

What to Do

Exhale completely and begin to observe the cycles of inhalations and exhalations and the spaces in between. As you inhale, observe how the breath flows on both sides and dimensions of the body, not only the front. Notice how the air enters on the nasal cavity and travels through the back of the throat, trachea, upper lobe, middle lobe, and lower lobes (bronchi) of the right lung and upper and lower bronchi of the left side. The ribs expand from inside out, and the breath becomes deeper and spreads from the capillaries of the lungs to the blood that carries it to the heart and nourishes the cells. As you exhale, the air moves back in reverse order. In each breathing cycle, the pelvic, thoracic, and chest diaphragms move like a cylinder, as the breath brings sensation to the entire trunk. In each inhalation, there is a sense of expansion, and on each exhalation, the expansion continues and creates a sensation of infinitude and space deep within as the diaphragm and abdominal organs soften. As you inhale, soften the belly as you feel the expansion of the inhalations and how it can support the convex ribs or the areas that drop. As you exhale, let the outgoing breath elongate and move the concave ribs out. On the next inhalation, let go of any tracking and let the breath permeate both sides and throughout the entire body. Rest as long as you need. To come out, roll to the right side and come away from the props. Press your left hand down, and, keeping the gaze down, come to a sitting position—the head is last to come up.

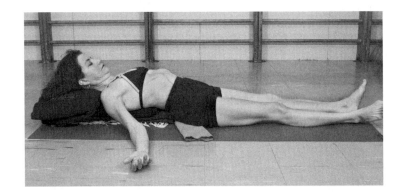

CHAIR

Note

In the breathing practices of yoga (pranaya-ma), breath is always through the nose, with exceptions related to one's health.

Sitting positions are very challenging with any structural pathology. The chair can provide stability for the trunk, and improve posture. If the position of the legs inside of the chair is too restricted, straddle the legs as shown in the second and third photos. The closer positioning of the legs will offer a compacted position and reference the midline, while the straddle position releases the back muscles, provides the space and stability for the sides to adjust, and softens the abdominal and pelvic organs while the spine elongates. If the feet do not reach the floor, place the blocks under the feet. Bring attention to the pelvic floor, the first vertebra of the sacrum, first lumbar vertebra, the 90 thoracic vertebrae, and the center of the breastbone.

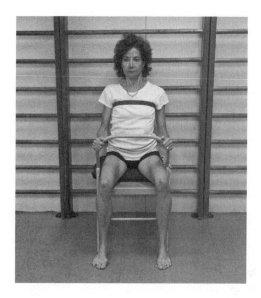

Placement

Sit facing the back of the chair, with the legs inside or around the backrest. The feet are parallel, and the lower leg establishes a perpendicular angle. The shoulders and arms are relaxed. Observe the sitting bones; see if one tends to carry more weight. Use a pad under the side that feels light. Hold the back of the chair, with the forearms parallel to the floor, but relaxed. Bring the shoulder blades in and lift the middle of the chest bone. The sacrum moves slightly in and the lumbar spine lifts up. On the concave side, add extra pressure and weight on the upper thigh; you can place a sandbag on that thigh. As the legs ground, the hips compact and the spine lifts. Lift the chest and use the hands and arms to compact the convex ribs and lift the concave. Slowly lift the chest bone, spread the clavicles, move the last cervical vertebra (C7) in, and lower the back of the head toward the chest.

What to Do

Ground the feet, compact the hips, and spread the sitting bones. Move the top of the sacrum in and ascend the pubic bone. Pull the hands down, roll the shoulders back, and the outer shoulder blade in, as the chest bone lifts and the head lowers. Observe the cycles of inhalations, exhalations, and the pauses in between for a few seconds. Bring the head up and rest.

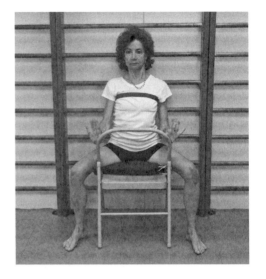

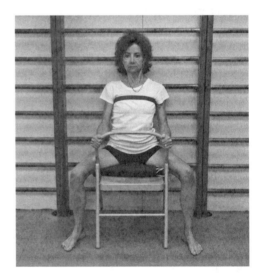

FINAL SAVASANA

Benefits

The removal of the props allows for the discovery of the body's natural state and offers insight into what can be done to adjust and improve alignment.

Props

Mat, blanket.

Lie in savasana without props, just a blanket under the head. Sometimes, it is important to feel one's own structure and inner support. Surrender the efforts and trust the support of the earth, softening the areas that move away and lifting the areas that collapse. The breath spreads and equalizes the tone of the whole body.

PART
III

ON DAILY LIFE

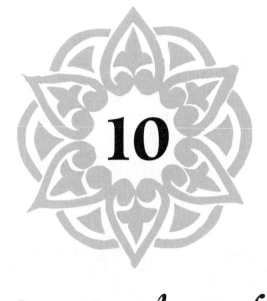

10

On Daily Life

The second chapter of Patanjali's *Yoga Sutras*, Sadhana Pada (Sutra 11.33), states: *Vitarkabadhane pratipaksabhavanam*, that is "Through discrimination, the obstacles that prevent one's evolution are to be countered by the opposing action." Principles that are countered by the yamas and niyamas are to be countered with the knowledge of discrimination.[1]

This chapter offers ways to work with scoliosis in daily life. Many of the suggestions will seem like the opposite to what feels natural and familiar. The idea is to develop and sustain a discriminating mind that can perceive the action of the body and its habits, and offer new and healthier choices. Study yourself daily. Get to know your habits, what feels comfortable and habitual, and what feels different and, perhaps, not so comfortable but, on the overall, more organized. Using the principle of nonviolence, we become our own best friend with discrimination.

WHAT TO OBSERVE

Which side bears the weight when lying, sitting, standing, and walking? Shift to the opposing side and distribute the weight evenly. Which side of the head tends to tilt? Try the opposite side, the nonhabitual, and then bring it to center by lifting the upper lobes of the ears up. Which ear and eye is the most active in daily functional life, such as when you are conversing with others or reading a book? Are your speech and words integrated with what you feel? On which side of the mouth do you often chew? Notice how you hold the utensils.

Sleeping

How do you sleep? On which side do you sleep? Which side is uncomfortable? Do you lie on your belly or your back? How is the position of your limbs? Observe which side you tend to sleep on, and then move to the opposite side. Change your position on the bed as well. Observe if your position brings compression or decompression of the spine.

Is your mattress soft or hard? It is important to buy a good quality mattress. It should be firm and without undulations. Notice what pillows you use, their height, and quality. Do research on special therapeutic mattresses and pillows. Consult your physical therapist or physician to recommend the proper support during your sleep.

Thinking

Choosing a healthier "neuro-pathway" of your ingrained habits, including your thoughts, is possible through consistent practice. For instance, what kinds of thought patterns occur when you are facing obstacles and when there is fatigue? Does the spine become more asymmetric? Try to feel when you collapse, tilt, and become unstable; how does it reflect on the physical, mental, and emotional body. These extra tilts and collapses shift the energetic channels from within and cause further imbalances. When having disturbing thought patterns, work with the yoga principle of choosing opposing thoughts.

Going against the grain of one's tendencies for a healthier life begins with observation that will lead to awareness so new habits can be integrated.

Sitting

The pelvis is the fulcrum of your seated posture. Observe how you sit. Which side of your pelvis receives more weight? Shift to the other side. Are you sitting on your tail bone and rounding the spine? Which side do you tend to lean toward? Lean to the other side. Where is the rotational direction of each side? Rotate to the opposite side. The proper distribution of weight and correction of the pelvis will depend on the nature of individual scoliosis, lumbar curve, or compensation. Where is the rotational direction of your pelvis?

How do the feet rest on the floor? The feet should rest on the floor about a hip-width apart, with the "eye" of the knees facing front and over the ankle joint. The groin can be released by elevating the pelvis with a support. When sitting, the feet are even, as in Tadasana, with equal weight and balance between the inner and outer edges, the first and fifth metatarsals, and the heels. Look at your feet and make sure that one foot does not go forward or supinate (roll out), or move away from the midline (abduction). The feet reflect the spinal asymmetry, so we can address symmetry from the feet to the spine. For instance, the fixation of both feet with extra pressure on the right foot will help address counter-rotation in the left lumbar curve. The outer rotators of the hip stabilize the pelvis. Do not cross your legs. Usually, the habit of crossing the legs is a reflection of the lumbar curves and pelvic rotation. Inhibit the pattern and cross the opposite leg.

As mentioned in the sitting chapters, the pelvic floor consists of the two sitting bones—the tailbone (coccyx) and the pubic bone. It forms a triangular shape and supports the spine. Ideally, the pelvic floor spreads evenly. Both sitting bones should bear even weight. If the lower spine is collapsed (rounded), this is an indicator of fatigue and that you should increase the height of your seat with a cushion, phone book, or blankets, so the lumbar spine can find its anatomical curve and lift. The proper correction for the pelvis and proper support will depend on the individual curve.

Sitting is a huge challenge for those of us with scoliosis. Avoid sitting for long periods. For those working in front of a computer or at a desk, avoid being static. Get up and move around. Stretch and take pauses. Look for a proper chair for sitting and a support for the computer so that the screen is at eye level.

Once you learn about your curves and habitual posture, use the appropriate prop to support your sitting. Use a bolster, firm pillow, or therapeutic ball to support the whole back. The back should be supported and upright so the shoulders and arms can hang relaxed from the shoulder joints. If breathing is not full while seated, this indicates a collapsed posture.

Blocks can be placed on either side of the back, between the shoulder blades and the spine, so both sides will feel supported. Place a block underneath the armpit of the side that collapses, and move the ribs toward the block. If the feet do not touch the ground, place a phone book or some blocks under them. Support results in an effortless posture.

When fatigue comes, it is the red flag for you to stop what you are doing, stand up, and stretch. We need to become aware of these inner signals. Observe how fatigue reflects on breathing and on posture. Be aware of compensations from areas that overwork to sustain the posture. Use your improvised props to facilitate stability and length.

Because of my long hours at the computer, I use all the props mentioned earlier, including a pad under one sitting bone to even and bring proper weight distribution. The principle is to position the belt on the apex of the curves, with the proper pad support to constrain collapses caused by poor posture. Do not tighten the belt too much, for it will affect breathing. There should be space between the skin and the belt so breathing can permeate.

One strategy for sitting that makes the position comfortable is to place weight on the upper thighs; this releases the legs from the pelvis. This action will ground the bones and the hip flexors and offer space for the spine to lengthen.

When traveling long distances, such as on international flights, bring small soft balls (such as those found in physiotherapy stores) to prop and massage the back, and small pillows as well. Change sitting positions often. Move and stretch the body. In the back of the plane there is room to stretch and do yoga.

Walking

The worst thing for the spine is a bad shoe, and the worst of all are high-heeled shoes. It is important to invest in good shoes that will provide support for the arches and offer resilience to the gait so the feet are flexible and supported.

Study your gait when walking on the street and climbing stairs. Observe which leg initiates the movement. Which leg internally rotates or externally rotates? Which leg is agile, and which one is slow? It is my experience that the slower leg side is the concave side, needing more attention and education to become expressive. The stronger side of the scoliosis can teach the weaker one. This has been a lesson received from my teacher Mr. Iyengar. Begin walking with the noninitiating side. Healthy joints move with ease and have rhythm. The transfer of weight is done from the center of the heels to the toes. Walk forward, backward, and sideways to increase spatial proprioception.

Carrying Objects

When you need to carry a handbag or shopping bag, use a backpack instead, so the weight is distributed and the thoracic diaphragm does not drop. Avoid carrying things on one side. For instance, if the convex side is the one that is initiating movement and carrying weight, use the opposite side instead. Although the muscles of the concave side are weaker, it is important to distribute the weight between both sides. Mothers often ask what to do for kids who carry schoolbooks. The backpack is a good solution; if this is not possible, shift the weight to different sides so the scoliosis is not aggravated.

To pick up a weight, bring the object closer to the center of the body instead of to the side, and use the legs and arms to lift with a neutral spine (maintaining the integrity of the four natural curves). Instead of compressing the spine, lengthen it. Lastly, ask for help if the weight is too much to bear.

Water Exercise

In ancient Greece, philosophers such as Thales and Democritus reflected on the importance of water. Thales believed that the one essential reality is water. He also believed that the earth floated on water; that all things were made of water; and that water is filled with God.

Swimming is a great gift in the healing journey of scoliosis. The water has the power to soothe the overworked muscles and add space and breadth to the compressed side. The lack of gravity is pure freedom for an asymmetric shape. It is the best therapeutic sport for skeletal muscle pathologies, for the respiratory system, and, most of all, for the mind. When we swim, we breathe and release the asymmetric form.

Organization

Organizing one's life can be a challenge when dealing with asymmetries. The reeducation to make things symmetrical happens in the external environment as well. The important thing is to bring the external environment into order with the organization of time, daily tasks, and household, personal, and business life.

Start with the yoga props and organize them in one corner. After practicing, place everything back so you can start anew. Organization with the environment is important and creates a constraint from which the nervous system can learn how to find order and center.

The Future Is the Present

Begin from where you are. Begin a yoga program under the guidance of a qualified teacher, along with support from good physicians, therapists, family, friends, and, most important of all, yourself. Understand that there will be distractions and obstacles on the path. It is important to work on the principle of repetition, sustained practice, curiosity of learning, and detachment. The following is one of my favorite verses from *The Bhagavadgita*:

"Progress on the path to perfection is slow and one may have to tread through many lives before reaching the end. But no effort is wasted. The relations we form and the powers we acquire do not perish at death. They will be the starting point for later development."[2]

REFERENCES

1. Iyengar, B. K. S. (2005). *Light on the Yoga Sutras of Patanjali*. New Delhi, India: APH Publishing.
2. Radhakrishnan, S. (1973). *The Bhagavadgītā*. Comment by the author on Verse 43. New York: HarperCollins.

Appendix

ADDITIONAL EXERCISES

This section suggests movements that are not asana-based that I find can enhance the repertoire of possibilities to help scoliosis.

SPINAL TRACTION

Props

Wall, pull-up bars.

Benefits

The hanging position lengthens both sides of the spine and the vertical diameter of the trunk as it creates space for the organs.

Placement

Reach and hold the upper bars of the support; the arms are alongside the ears. Observe if one arm is closer to the ear than the other. Spread the arms accordingly (decentralize) to create space between the neck and shoulders.

What to Do

As both hands grasp the bar, pull and rotate the upper arms, move the shoulders away from the ears, and bring the outer edges (lateral angle) of the shoulder blades in and down. Compact the convex ribs in and move the concave ribs out. Stretch the legs away from your arms and bring the abdomen in.

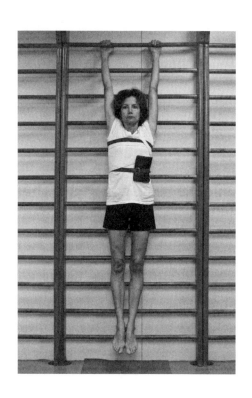

For Lumbar Curve

Further reach your feet down as you pull the arms; lift the ribs up and away from the hip as the spine moves in and the chest opens.

Caution

Do not let the body weight collapse because doing so will harm your ligaments.

ILIOPSOAS MUSCLES RELEASE

Props

Wall, block.

Benefit

Releases the psoas major, separates the leg from the trunk, and elongates the lumbar spine.

What to Do

Stand with your right side adjacent to the wall. Place a block under the left foot; the leg nearest to the wall is free to gently swing like a pendulum. Place your right arm on the wall and begin to crawl up the wall with the fingers of the right hand. For right thoracic scoliosis, the right hand can press on the wall so the top of the arm (head of humerus) moves into the socket, and the outer shoulder blade wraps in and stabilizes toward the spine. Begin to add an up-and-down motion to release the leg from the waist and the hip from the rib. Keep the standing leg as in tasadana (long and firm), and compact both outer hips in from the action of the lateral rotators (outer hip).

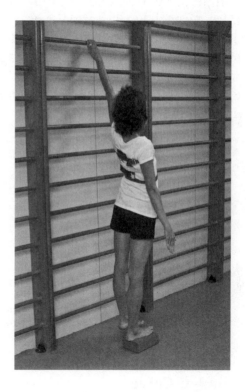

Change sides. Stand with your left side facing the wall (as shown in the photo). Step onto the block with your right foot as the left leg hangs. Press down with the right foot and lift the left leg up; the outer hip moves in as the left leg swings like a pendulum from front to back. Begin to crawl up the wall with the fingers of the left hand to lengthen the left side. As the left leg moves like a pendulum, the ribs move away from the pelvis and toward the wall.

If the left side is the concave side, the left ilium is lifted from the chronic muscular holding of the quadratus lumborum fibers (extend lateral flexes and rotate the spine). Hold the position longer on this side, and with micro movements, release the leg and climb the fingers of the left hand up the wall.

Note

You can perceive the same action in climbing stairs. As each leg lifts and flexes, notice how it relates to the lumbar spine and how one side is shorter and harder. The goal in this sequence is to start the movement from the leg of the retracted side and to separate the leg from the trunk.

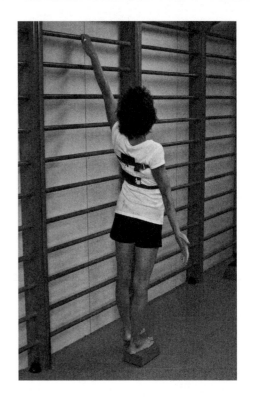

OPENING THE LUNGS

Props

Mat, bolster.

Benefits

Massages and opens the lobes of the lungs.

Placement

Lie on your right side, with the right ribs facing a horizontal bolster. The right side of the head is supported by a folded blanket. The left arm is over the ear. The legs are extended.

What to Do

Observe the breath in the left lung. Gradually breathe in segmentally from the lower portion of the lung to the upper. Rest. Change sides.

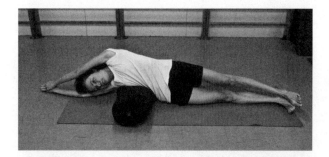

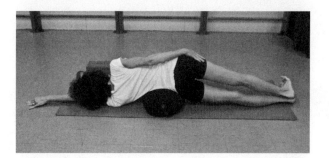

Variation 1

Lie prone, with the belly on the bolster. Inhale into the concave side and exhale from the convex side. Rest. Breathe normally.

Variation 2

Lie with the middle chest on the bolster and the head supported on a blanket. Inhale into the concave side and exhale from the convex. Rest. Breathe normally.

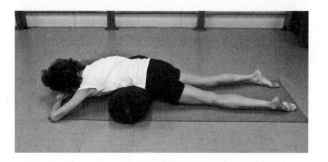

GAIT

Walking is the most basic human activity, and it starts when we are babies, exploring the environment and becoming independent. Likewise, yoga teaches us how to explore our relationship to the world to become self-reliant and free.

Walking is a functional and daily activity, and with asymmetries it can feel like a challenging task. As we learn how to properly align and use the legs to perform their function for locomotion, walking becomes lighter and less energy is spent. One important key to achieving a more efficient walk is to use the eyes to maintain the upright posture. As the eyes look down, the spine sags, and vice versa. The lift of the trunk is organized by the postural and abdominal muscles, while the nose, the center of the sternum, the navel, and the pubic bone act as a reference for midline and center.

Studying Your Gait

Walk across the room and observe both sides.

Things to Observe

Which leg moves faster? How is the weight distributed from the heel to the metatarsus? Does one side receive more weight? Does one leg feel freer or lighter? Does one hip rotate more than the other? How does each arm swing?

Variation 1

Now, as you walk, let the heel touch the floor first, then extend the toes. Extend both arms down and reach with the fingers toward the floor. Roll the shoulders back, move the outer edges of the shoulder blades in, lift both sides of the rib cage, slightly lift the pubic bone up, and compact. Both of your eyes look to the front. The tops of the ears should be parallel and the head in line with the spine. Add speed to this walk.

Variation 2

Repeat the walk, reaching down with both arms, and lower the shoulders away from your ears. Now, add the lift of each leg as you walk forward, keeping the hips in line, the heel-first stride, and the extension of the toes.

Variation 3

A more challenging way to enhance proprioception of the back is to walk backward. Imagine that the back has eyes. While walking backward, maintain a front-facing gaze while the crown of the head stays up. The toes should touch the floor first, then the heels.

Benefits

Increases proprioception and balance.

Resources

ORGANIZATIONS

International Society on Scoliosis Orthopaedic and Rehabilitation Treatment: http://www
.fixscoliosis.com/threads/4-SOSORT-%28Society-on-Scoliosis-Orthopaedic-and-
Rehabilitation-Treatment%29

RECOMMENDED READING: ANATOMY AND SOMATIC STUDIES

Cassella, Michelina C., and John E. Hall. "Current Treatment Approaches in the Nonoperative
and Operative Management of Adolescent Idiopathic Scoliosis." *Physical Therapy* 71,
no. 12 (1991): 897–909.

Cochard, Larry R. *Netter's Atlas of Human Embryology*. Philadelphia: Saunders, 2002.

Cohen, Bonnie Bainbridge. *Sensing, Feeling, and Action: The Experiential Anatomy of
Body–Mind Centering*. Northampton, MA: Contact Editions, 1993.

Feldenkrais, Moshe. *Awareness Through Movement: Easy-to-do Health Exercises to Improve
Your Posture, Vision, Imagination, and Personal Awareness*. New York: Harper One, 1991.

Fiorentino, Mary R. *A Basis for Sensorimotor Development—Normal and Abnormal: The
Influence of Primitive, Postural Reflexes on the Development and Distribution of Tone*.
Springfield, IL: Charles C. Thomas, 1981.

Hawes, Martha. *Scoliosis and The Human Spine*. Tuscon, AZ: Willowship Press, 2002.

Netter, Frank H. *Atlas of Human Anatomy*. 5th ed. Philadelphia: Saunders, 2010.

Perdriolle, René. *La Scoliose: Son Étude Tridimensionnelle*. Paris: Maloine S.A. Editeur, 1979.

RECOMMENDED READING: YOGA STUDIES

Gandhi, Mahatma. *The Bhagavad Gita According to Gandhi*. Berkeley, CA: North Atlantic Books, 2009.

Iyengar, B. K. S. *Light on Life*. New York: Rodale, 2005.

Iyengar, B. K. S. *Light on Pranayama: The Yogic Art of Breathing*. New York: Crossroad Publishing, 1985.

Iyengar, B. K. S. *Light on the Yoga Sutras of Patanjali*. New Delhi, India: APH Publishing, 2005.

Iyengar, B. K. S. *Light on Yoga: The Bible of Modern Yoga*. New York: Schocken Books, 1995.

Iyengar, Geeta. *Yoga: A Gem for Women*. Kootenay, Canada: Timeless Books, 2002.

Iyengar, Geeta. *Yoga in Action: Preliminary Course*. Mumbai, India: Highflown Advertising, 2000.

Iyengar, Prashant. *The Alpha and Omega of Trikonasana*. Mumbai, India: Iyengar Yogashraya, 2004.

Radhakrishnan, S. *The Bhagavadgītā*. New York: HarperCollins, 1973.

Swatmarama, Swami. *Hatha Yoga Pradipika: Sanskrit and English*. Forgotten Books, 2008.

Index

Note: Boldface numbers indicate illustrations